Survival Skills for GPs

Ruth Chambers

General Practitioner
Professor of Health Commissioning
School of Health
Staffordshire University

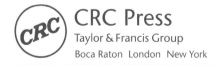

CRC Press
Taylor & Francis Group
Boca Raton London New York

CRC Press is an imprint of the
Taylor & Francis Group, an **informa** business

Illustrations © 1999 Martin Davies

CRC Press
Taylor & Francis Group
6000 Broken Sound Parkway NW, Suite 300
Boca Raton, FL 33487-2742

Printed on acid-free paper
Version Date: 20150924

International Standard Book Number-13: 978-1-85775-334-9 (Paperback)

Visit the Taylor & Francis Web site at
http://www.taylorandfrancis.com

and the CRC Press Web site at
http://www.crcpress.com

CONTENTS

CONTENTS

PREFACE

General practice is no longer the job it once was. GPs have progressed from paper and pen to computers and information technology, from isolated single-handed practices to supportive partnerships, from relative autonomy to team work. In theory, these changes and many others resulting from the restructuring of primary care and the NHS should make the working conditions for GPs and their practice team easier. There are more effective treatments, other health professionals with whom to share the workload, information and evidence about best practice literally at your finger tips on the keyboard, practice managers to take on responsibility for the organisational side of general practice, and a shift from home visiting to surgery consultations.

But changes which are immense, swift and sometimes imposed, typically result in stress and turmoil for the individuals concerned. The gradual erosion of their autonomy has been stressful for many GPs who were used to being in control of their own working practices before guidelines or audit were in vogue, let alone before clinical governance was thought of. Loss of control is one of the three main components of stress, the other two parts being lack of support and high demands, both of which are usual features of today's general practice team.

Survival is not only about learning to cope with the changed circumstances of general practice but how to flourish and enjoy your working life. That is why this book takes you the reader on a path from becoming more aware of what is causing you stress at work and home, the effects of stress on you and how you usually react to it (Module 1), to looking at ways of enhancing your career and developing yourself further as a person and as a professional (Module 6). The intervening sections starting with Module 2 increase your understanding of the range of options and solutions that are available to you to control stress or minimise it if you cannot obliterate it completely. You are encouraged to practise being more assertive and to manage your time better in Modules 3 and 4 as these are two key skills which will help you to control your workload in a pro-active way, and create more time for your own interests.

Understanding more about what gives you job satisfaction in Module 5 and how you might increase it should help to make you more resilient to change, stress, or adverse life events. You need to develop skills that are integral to you, that will help you handle any significant stress, change, or adverse life events that come your way. Your more highly developed personal and professional satisfaction should be a positive force that protects you in years to come from disillusionment and low morale.

The six Modules make up the *Survival Skills* programme for GPs. They have evolved from the popular long distance learning programme written as part of the Stress Fellowship of the Royal College of General Practitioners. The original programme was approved for 24 hours postgraduate educational accreditation by the national panel. A time allotment has been calculated for each Module here to guide the reader as to how long it should take to read and reflect on the relevance of each Module for their situation and complete the exercises. You should be able to apply for one or all Modules to be approved by your local Deanery for self-directed study with the agreement and support of your GP tutor who may be willing to provide feedback. It will be better still if your local GP tutor organises a small group of GPs to undertake the *Survival Skills* programme together. Primary care groups might encourage peer groups of GPs to work through the programme in the same way. You might take your time and undertake one Module every few months or complete them all straight after each other in a relatively short time. The beauty of a programme like this is that you can work at your own pace.

This *Survival Skills* programme should remind you of the many strengths and opportunities you already have. Following the programme should build up your confidence in your own personal and professional qualities so that by the end of the sixth Module you will agree that general practice is no longer the job it was – it is better!

Ruth Chambers
April 1999

To my family, Steph, Rob, Dave and Chris who have relieved more stress
than they have provoked (just!)

MODULE 1
Detecting symptoms and causes of stress

AIMS

The aims of Module 1 are:

1 To help GPs become more aware of the causes of stress in themselves and others.

2 To help GPs appreciate the effects of stress on themselves and others.

3 To help GPs realise the impact of adverse stress on their work.

CONTENTS

What is stress?

Symptoms of stress
Exercise 1: What symptoms of stress are you suffering?
(time = 20 mins)

Causes of stress
Exercise 2: Compare your causes of stress with other people's views
(time = 20 mins)
Exercise 3: Review your own personality type (time = 20 mins)
Exercise 4: Complete a series of daily logs to check whether you have identified all your causes of stress (time = 5 hours)

Effects of stress
Exercise 5: Draw your own stress performance curve (time = 15 mins)
Exercise 6: Compare the effects you perceive that stress has on you with what others think about themselves (time = 20 mins)
Exercise 7: Summarising sources and effects of stress for you
(time = 40 mins)
Exercise 8: Are you experiencing too much stress? Do you need help? Making changes (time = 30 mins)

The total time to work through the module depends on the amount of time the reader spends reflecting on how the information in the module applies to him or her, before completing the exercises. The total time for which postgraduate education accreditation might be sought is nine hours (including time for reading and thinking and so long as 10 days' worth of stress logs are completed).*

---

* GP participants could apply to their region's Director of Postgraduate General Practice Education for permission to submit one or more completed modules for postgraduate education accreditation. Approval of such an application will be at the Director's discretion and may require the support of a local GP tutor in arranging assessment. No assessment will be undertaken by the author or Radcliffe Medical Press.

Here's what some GP participants said they had gained from undertaking the first *Survival Skills for GPs* programme:

'The programme made me realise I am not alone and that there are changes I can make to improve some of my stress problems.'

'Doing the Survival Skills programme yourself makes you think more than attending a course would.'

'I had hoped that someone would know more than I did about dealing with stress but then it was reassuring to know that I did know as much as anyone else on the subject. It made me stop and consider the problems and organisation of the practice and realise that we are actually doing quite well.'

'It was stimulating and enlightened sensitive issues.'

'I enjoyed looking more closely at different aspects of my working life, how I feel about it, and what could be improved.'

'Having to analyse my individual day was very helpful.'

'Especially good parts were … breaking down areas of stress into manageable bits … took me in stages through my stressors … could be tackled where and when wanted which was very helpful.'

'The programme allowed me to think about the events and effects on everyone involved.'

'It helped me to look at the good points of my work.'

'It helps to understand stress and reactions of the body so that you can apply the understanding and minimise the effects.'

'Useful to see how much of my stress equalled other GPs', as so much of it is inherent in the job.'

'Makes you think about your life.'

'It encourages self-analysis and a "confessional" spirit to admit "sins" of self-destruction.'

'Having to write down information ensures excellent concentration.'

'I liked the effective content and approach to creating change in my life.'

WHAT IS STRESS?

Stress is very difficult to define as it is such a vague word and everyone interprets it differently. Stress is equivalent to a person's perception of the pressure upon them, or the 'three way relationship between demands on a person, that person's feelings about those demands and their ability to cope with those demands'.[1] So, in other words, a particular event or task can be very stressful for you one day but not on another, all depending on how you are feeling and what other pressures are being exerted on you.

In general, stress occurs in situations where the workload is high, control over the workload is limited and too little is available in the way of support or help. Many GPs would say they know when they're feeling stressed even if they cannot specify exactly what stress is!

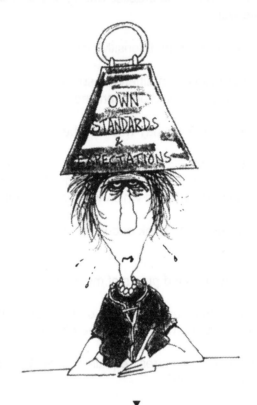

▼

What is stress?

Is stress bad for you? It depends on how much stress you are under, how long it is applied for, whether you feel powerless to stand up to the stress or can overcome it. Certainly a moderate amount of stress is necessary to perform well at work and to maintain a zest for life; zero stress may lead to boredom whereas too much stress over too long a period will render you indecisive, exhausted or burnt out.

Are GPs 'special cases' in suffering from stress? Stress affects the whole of today's society; doctors are not unique in reporting escalating levels of stress and low morale. In a typical week one million of the 24 million in the UK's labour force took one day off work and up to 40% of absenteeism is thought to be due to mental or emotional problems. But in medicine, caring for others creates additional stresses from daily exposure to human distress and ill health, and the daily striving for perfection in relieving all suffering and never making mistakes.

Is stress an integral part of the job? It is important to distinguish between an occasional event or task that creates the highest levels of stress and those that cause the most frequent reports of stress. For example, an official complaint by a patient might cause terrific stress but hopefully rarely happens, whereas inappropriate requests for home visits may be a frequent cause of stress. A steady, relentless drip, drip, drip of stress-provoking situations may be just as likely to create a stressed doctor as a crisis event with monumental stress attached.

Surveys of doctors describe such a range of causes of stress that it seems as if the list of stressors is just the ingredients of daily life that make up the job description of a general practitioner! In other words, almost everything GPs do as part of their work has the potential to create stress in some people, depending on the quantity and quality of that source of pressure.

The sort of things that GPs describe *most commonly* as causing them to feel stressed are:

- demands of the job
- patients' inappropriate expectations
- interruptions
- practice administration
- the conflict at the work–home interface between career and family
- interference with social life
- dealing with death and dying.

Female GPs experience more stress than their male colleagues from home visiting, fear of assault, finding a locum, the working environment, lack of emotional support at home and dealing with friends or relatives as patients.

The stressors that cause the *highest levels* of stress have been described by GPs as being:

- relationship conflicts with other doctors
- making mistakes
- conflict of career with family life
- fear of litigation
- work/demand overload.

The main way of identifying what provokes stress in you is to become more aware when symptoms of stress occur. Doctors are well known for denying that they themselves suffer stress or other ill-health symptoms, as they perceive such symptoms to be signs of weakness (or sometimes serious illness or even madness!). So the only way that you are going to understand how stress is affecting you, and through you others around you at work and home, is by identifying the sources, effects and consequent outcomes for yourself, and not just by reading books like this one. The next section starts to look at symptoms of stress. Over time you should come to realise which are most applicable to you.

SYMPTOMS OF STRESS

Stress at work does not happen in a vacuum. Pressures and problems at home often overflow on to how someone feels and performs at work, and the effects of stress at work are often taken home and unfairly dumped there. Different people suffer various proportions and mixes of physical, mental, emotional and behavioural types of symptoms.

Stress can affect everyone. It often goes undetected or unacknowledged by the sufferer him or herself. They may have been warned by others to 'slow down' and have delighted in ignoring such advice and pushing themselves on regardless. It is often people with 'Type A' personalities who react like this, and their particular characteristics will be explored a bit later.

EXERCISE 1   What symptoms of stress are you suffering?

Look at the list below of behavioural and personal symptoms described by people suffering from stress at work. Tick the ones you have experienced. When did you experience this? Recently or in the past? Changes in feelings or behaviour may well indicate stress.

How many are significant symptoms of stress for you or are they really quite trivial and unimportant? Circle the three most significant behavioural symptoms and the three most significant personal symptoms for you in the table below.

Behavioural symptoms	Tick the ones you have experienced	When did you experience this?
Lost confidence Shy away from paperwork Put things off Indecisive Shunt work away Working all weekends Underperforming Less efficient Late for work Longer working but less done Breakdown in relationships Argumentative Irritable Accident prone Loss of interest in sex Overeating Withdrawal from relationships		

Continued

Detecting symptoms and causes of stress

EXERCISE 1   Continued.

Personal symptoms	Tick the ones you have experienced	When did you experience this?
Anxious Palpitations Feeling burdened Insomnia Panic/hyperventilate Reduced appetite Tired/drained Jumpy Difficulty concentrating Depressed Nausea/indigestion Cynical Loss of confidence Lack of self-esteem Feelings of helplessness		

CAUSES OF STRESS

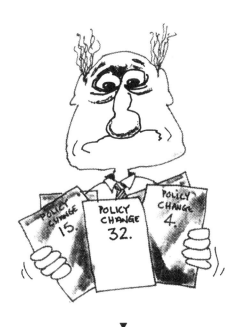

▼

Change and turmoil.

EXERCISE 2 Compare your causes of stress with others'.

To find out whether these causes of stress apply to you, fill in the questionnaire below about what causes *you* stress at work. The causes of stress are not in any order of priority. They have been identified by some GPs and practice managers as causes of stress at work for staff.[2] Tick whether these are sources of stress for you, ticking 'No stress', 'Somewhat' and 'Very stressful' according to how you perceive that factor. At the same time, rank each factor according to how important a stress it is for you, from 1 to 10 where '1' is the most important source of stress for you and '10' is the least important.

Stressor	No stress	Somewhat	Very stressful	Ranking
Lack of staff training				
Availability of appointments				
Paperwork				
Government policies				
Evidence-based guidelines				
Patient abuse or aggression				
Too much work				
Arguments and disputes between staff				
Patient demands				
Complaints				
Home visits				
Job insecurity				
Pay level				
GP demands on staff				
Long hours of work				
Antisocial working hours				
Poor communication				
Standard of workplace environment				
Other: (complete yours)				

Continued

Detecting symptoms and causes of stress

EXERCISE 2   Continued.

The study of GPs and practice managers found that they described the same six top causes of stress for staff. How did your ranking compare with theirs?

Please complete the third column to show how your answers compared with the published reports of other GPs and practice managers. Rank your top six; add any of your top causes of stress at the bottom of the table in the 'Other' rows to display your top six. If you are different from the average GP or practice manager think why. Is it because you are unaware that certain factors cause you stress or are your circumstances different?

Sources of stress	GPs' rank order	Practice managers' rank order	Your rank order
Patient demands	1	1	
Too much work	2	2	
Patient abuse/aggression	3	3	
Availability of appointments	4	4	
GP demands on staff	5	5	
Poor communication	6	6	
Other:			
Other:			
Other:			
Other:			
Other:			

Type A personality

GPs have a tendency to personality types which are more susceptible to stress. There is research to show that some doctors were attracted to medicine to seek the love and/or praise that were missing in their own childhoods. This make-up in their personality makes them more vulnerable to stress if they are constantly trying to please other people and are unduly upset by criticism or failure to meet high standards. Many doctors fit the 'Type A' personality picture; people with Type A characteristics are thought to be highly demanding of themselves and others, driving themselves to be perfectionists.

Type A behaviour is often learned in childhood, especially when the child strove to achieve to counteract low self-esteem or self-worth. Although some busy professionals may believe that Type A characteristics are a positive benefit in that they help them to get through their work quickly, in the longer term these characteristics are self-destructive. Type B personalities can be just as successful and achieve just as much as Type A personalities at a slower but steady pace. Type A behaviour can be modified with practice.

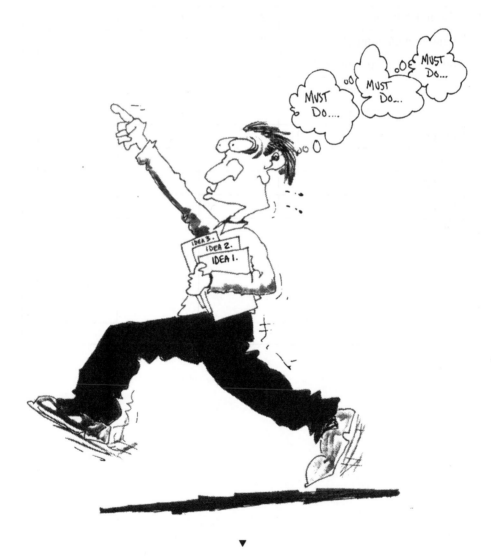

▼

Type A personality.

EXERCISE 3   Review your own personality type.

Please read through the list below and tick those factors which you feel correspond to your own personality. Now rate how extreme you feel you are for each Type A characteristic listed below out of a maximum score of '10', e.g. if you think that your feelings are absolutely contained score '10' in that column, or alternatively if you are very expressive of your feelings score '1'. Tick which factors you think encourage you to become over-stressed?

Type A characteristics	Rate factors as applied to you (score 1–10)	Which factors encourage stress in you?
Highly competitive		
Hard driving		
Feelings contained		
Sets frequent deadlines		
Meticulous about details		
Does everything fast		
Ambitious		
Fidgety if kept waiting		
Intolerant of mistakes		
Does more than one task at a time		
Anticipates others in conversation		
Hard worker – few outside interests		
Feels angry/impatient in queues		
Feels responsible		
Aggressive		
High achiever		
Continual sense of time urgency		
Easily upset/angry over trivia		

Looking at the table of Type A characteristic scores, pick the three highest-scoring factors. Write down below which factors you have selected and what plan of action it might be possible to take to reduce each factor you have selected.

High-scoring Type A characteristic	Possible action
1	
2	
3	

EXERCISE 4   Complete a series of daily logs to check whether you have identified all your causes of stress comprehensively.

Make five photocopies of the unused form for monitoring stress at work. Fill one in each day for a typical week, recording any significant sources of stress and your usual reactions or responses (either good or bad). For example, a 'bad' response or behaviour might be that you drove your car too fast after a row with one of the practice team, or lost your temper inappropriately after a succession of interruptions to your work. A 'good' response or behaviour might be that you reorganised a practice procedure or discussed your concerns with others.

Recording five days' worth should make sure that you get a spread of busy and less-pressured days. At the end of the week review your recordings for all five days and write down your most common stressors at work and your usual responses on the summary log form which follows.

Then repeat the exercise completing stress logs for the time you spend outside work – at home or in other places or situations, during the weekend, or before and after the working day. Photocopy several days' worth of stress log forms. As before, record your usual responses to any stress caused over several days. Stresses at home and in the environment may be intermingled with stresses at work and it could be difficult to separate out exact causes and effects. Summarise the sources of home and environmental stressors and your usual responses on the summary log form which follows.

You could complete and monitor daily logs for both in work and outside work at the same time, but to do so may put you under too much pressure. If you are continually watching and analysing yourself all day long, you may get fed up with this exercise and chuck the whole lot away.

Keep at it! If you want a break, leave off doing the log for a day or two and start again later in the week, rather than stopping all together.

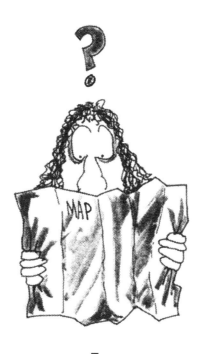

▼

Where are you now?

DAILY STRESS LOG AT WORK   Day and date: ....

Source of stress at work: My response:

....

....

....

....

....

....

....

....

....

....

....

....

....

....

Comments:

....

....

My overall stress level for today was:

0 1 2 3 4 5 6 7 8 9 10 (circle your reply)

DAILY STRESS LOG OUTSIDE WORK   Day and date: ....

Source of stress outside work: My response:

....

....

....

....

....

....

....

....

....

....

....

....

....

....

Comments:

....

....

My overall stress level for today was:

   0 1 2 3 4 5 6 7 8 9 10 (circle your reply)

SUMMARY STRESS LOG   **Overview of sources of stress and usual responses at work and outside work in week beginning:**

....

Most frequent sources of stress
at work:

My usual response:

....
....
....
....
....
....
....
....
....
....
....
....
....

Most frequent sources of stress
outside work:

My usual response:

....
....
....
....
....
....
....
....

There are other causes of stress in doctors and other health professionals that have not been referred to or explored yet in this workbook.

The mismatch and misfit of individuals for a career in the health field

Medical students are often selected for their academic attainments rather than their personal qualities. But society seems to want the sort of doctors who take time and trouble to listen and empathise. Unfortunately, doctors who have the highest empathy levels with patients when tested as students and young junior doctors, are the ones who 10 years later have the least contact time with patients. So, in other words, it seems as if they have not been able to sustain the emotionally draining good doctor–patient relationships at which they excel, except by reducing their general practice work and finding alternative sessional work outside family practice.

GPs and staff are often expected to conform to the traditional ways and styles of working of the practices they join. We should encourage doctors to dictate their own pace and styles at work and to encourage flexibility to suit their own particular circumstances. We know that doctors who are forced to work faster than the pace they prefer not only become stressed but also underperform.[3]

Caring for others

In medicine, caring for others creates additional stresses from daily exposure to human distress and ill health, from the desire to alleviate *all* suffering, and from striving to be perfect and never making mistakes.

Lack of a career structure in general practice

The lack of a clear career structure is a well-recognised cause of stress in any workforce, not just medicine. To gauge the importance of this stress in medicine we have to remember the type of people who entered medical school. They were the 'achievers' at school, the ones who gained the top marks in the examinations and had that 'something extra' to persuade those interviewing for medical school that they would 'make the grade' as doctors. After a decade of striving and commitment they enter general practice to find high service demands and, all at once, a seeming dead end to their career with no encouragement to continue studying and no recognition for improvements or further qualifications. General practitioner partners rarely support colleagues who want to do research or wish to have protected time to pursue educational interests. Extra academic activities have to be fitted in around heavy service commitments and commonly encroach on family or leisure time.

Lack of career choice, especially for women doctors

An additional stress for some women is that general practice may not have been their chosen career. Many leave the hospital specialty they would have preferred, such as paediatrics or obstetrics, because they could see that few women made it to the top and that the general practice lifestyle is more likely to be compatible with bringing up a family. Even when they have become GP principals there is inequality between the sexes, with male doctors continuing to manage the side of general practice looked upon as a traditionally masculine preserve, such as finance, computers and minor surgery, and female doctors concentrating on women's health in the practice.[4] If you are not working in your chosen career specialty you are less likely to find your job satisfying and more likely to be stressed. And career counselling for doctors or any other primary care health professionals is virtually non-existent. Many junior or established doctors have no idea where they might go to find information or practical help about part-time training, changing specialties or retraining for a different medical career.

Escalating workload

In the United Kingdom there has been a shift of patient care to general practice from the hospital sector without a proportionate increase in

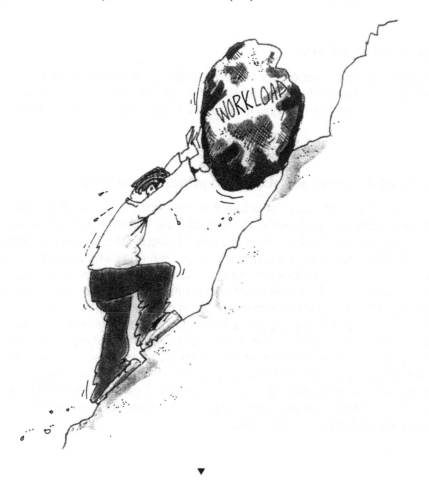

▼

Escalating workload.

resources. In addition, there has been a relative explosion of consumer demand and family doctors have extended their range of services. In some other countries where payment is according to the volume of work, doctors have coped with high workloads for some time. But those doctors have a degree of choice and control over that workload, whereas in Britain, family doctors have had little say in the continuing escalating workload.

It is easy to predict what happens when extra work is continually piled on to an already busy GP with little, if any, of the previous work being transferred away. For a while everything appears in order, the GP keeps going but works a little faster and appears, on the surface, to be coping. But gradually, in order to absorb the additional work, standards start to slide. There is a conflict between high performance targets and quantity of work: professional codes of practice and quality of work. As quality starts to slip, GPs may start to take short cuts, fail to do quite what's best for each patient or treat the psychosomatic symptoms a patient offers at face value instead of exploring the psychological basis and underlying distress, for example. The doctor feels guilty and dissatisfied and knows he or she could, should and used to practise better care. We know that the extent to which a doctor is self-critical is a strong predictor of stress, and when doctors are forced to deliver quantity rather than quality and drop their own high standards of care just to 'survive', they will be more self-critical and therefore more likely to be stressed. But it is not just a question of too much work. There is a direct relationship between lack or loss of control, work overload and stress. Stress reduction initiatives have either to reduce demands or increase participation in control, or preferably both.

Change and turmoil

Change and turmoil have bedevilled the health service over the last few years, as it has other professions and services too. Fundholding both created and solved stress as GPs were divided about whether they saw it as an additional stress or as a method to regain control and eventually reduce stress levels. Reorganisation of practices into primary care groups (PCGs) is bound to cause stress because of the uncertainty and extent of change involved, which has been compounded by the slow release of regulations concerning the structure and functioning of PCGs. Partnerships between organisations and the different health and social care disciplines have been much talked about, but may well create unacceptable tensions as professionals working closely with each other will have different employers, separate funding, varied terms and conditions, and dissimilar cultures.

Disturbing life events

GPs will have changes and adversity in their lives in the same way as anyone else does. These may concern relationships – marriage, divorce, bereavement, births, etc. – or changes in their circumstances, such as moving house, switching jobs or retirement.

EFFECTS OF STRESS

Effects of stress on general practice working

The potential human and organisational costs resulting from the consequences of excessively stressed doctors are enormous. Improving the mental health of doctors and other healthcare staff could increase the effectiveness of the whole organisation. Put simply, stress in doctors affects the quality of patient care, but it is a difficult message to drive home convincingly for individual doctors and NHS management.

Effects of stress in the workplace[5]

- Reduced productivity
- Lack of creativity
- Increased errors
- Poor decision making
- Job dissatisfaction
- Poor timekeeping
- Disloyalty
- Increased sick leave
- Increased complaints
- Premature retirement
- Absenteeism
- Accidents
- Thefts
- Organisational breakdown.

Translating these effects into the consequences of stress in primary care, you might consider that:

- Reduced productivity could lead to a stressed doctor's reluctance to explore patients' underlying problems and accepting psychosomatic symptoms at face value, or refusing to accommodate 'extra' patients on their surgery lists.

- Increased errors may be translated into mistakes in prescribing, administering drugs or any other part of patient care.

- Lack of creativity could mean less chance of innovative practice developments, and fewer options of care devised and offered to patients.

- Poor decision making may cause doctors to increase their referral and investigation rates when they feel unable to take responsibility for deciding about patients' likely diagnoses, as they are no longer able to live with the degree of uncertainty associated with making probable diagnoses as compared to definite diagnoses.

• Organisational breakdown may be demonstrated by inter-personal difficulties in the practice team, the extreme of which is partnership breakdown, an all too common event nowadays.

Stress and performance

There is a common misconception amongst doctors and NHS managers that there is a linear relationship between the extent of demands applied to individuals and their performance at work. Instead, there is an optimum level of demand where the individual is decisive, creative, working efficiently and effectively. After this point, if a sensible level of demand is exceeded performance tails off and the individual doctor becomes less effective, less decisive, etc., and eventually exhausted and burnt out. Figure 1 below illustrates this sequence of events. The fantasy line shown is the mental picture many doctors have of themselves.

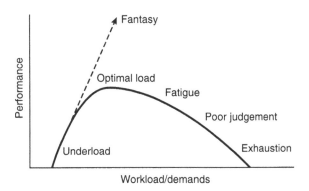

Figure 1: Stress performance curve.

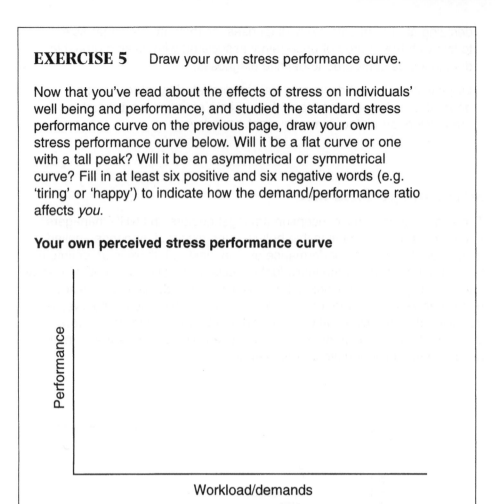

EXERCISE 5   Draw your own stress performance curve.

Now that you've read about the effects of stress on individuals' well being and performance, and studied the standard stress performance curve on the previous page, draw your own stress performance curve below. Will it be a flat curve or one with a tall peak? Will it be an asymmetrical or symmetrical curve? Fill in at least six positive and six negative words (e.g. 'tiring' or 'happy') to indicate how the demand/performance ratio affects *you*.

Your own perceived stress performance curve

Performance

Workload/demands

Effects of stress on individual GPs

The performance of stressed doctors will frequently be under par and the seriousness of the lapses may vary from slight errors or omissions to potentially fatal mistakes. In addition there is the possibility of stress litigation by doctors in the future against health service managers. Another cost to the organisation has been the loss of stressed doctors who have become too sick to continue at work. In the past, the medical profession has colluded with managers in 'medicalising' stress. It has traditionally been considered that a doctor who has been unable to work because of stress or depression long term has a primarily medical problem, rather than blaming their illness on poor management.

The most important consequence of the soaring stress levels in primary care is the high rate of mental health problems and low morale of GPs and their practice teams. The medical newspapers are full of the topic and this has led to the unjustified accusation by some that stress in doctors is exaggerated by the press and has created the situation rather than reported it. Studies report that around half of GPs may have borderline or be cases of anxiety, and about a quarter have borderline or be cases of depression.[6,7] This compares with similar rates for hospital consultants, whereas NHS managers had similar rates of anxiety but significantly lower rates of depression.

The effects of stress on individual health professionals will be evident as:

1 Individual symptoms, including changes in feelings, behaviour, thinking and well being, as have been covered earlier in this module.

2 Organisational symptoms, including all aspects of performance at work, and relationships with others at the practice and outside NHS bodies.

The effects of the stress 'virus' on partners and staff at work are:

1 Poor team spirit/work in the practice.

2 Breakdown in communication.

3 Too little time for each other so no deep bonds of friendship or regard are formed.

4 Too little support for each other.

5 Others feel stressed being in the company of the stressed health professional.

The effects of stress on those at home are:

1 Feeling that the stressed GP is disinterested so that family bonds deteriorate.

2 One problem creates another (marital or child's).

3 Lack of support and cohesion.

4 Children/wives feel they are unimportant compared to the stressed GP's work.

5 Breakdown of family unit.

6 Stressed GP is preoccupied.

EXERCISE 6   Compare the effects you perceive that stress has on you with what other GPs and practice managers think about themselves.

To find out whether these effects of stress apply to you, fill in the questionnaire below about what effects stress has on *you* at work. The effects of stress are not in any order of priority. They have been identified by some GPs and practice managers as effects of stress at work for them.[2] Tick whether these are effects of stress for you, ticking 'No', 'Somewhat' and 'Significant' according to how you perceive that effect. At the same time, rank each effect according to how significant an effect it is for you, from 1 to 10 where '1' is the most significant effect of stress for you and '10' is the least significant.

Effect of stress on your practice or work unit	No	Somewhat	Significant	Ranking
Increased staff turnover				
Thefts				
Mistakes				
Poor timekeeping				
Reduced productivity				
Increased staff sickness				
Organisational breakdown				
Arguments or angry outbursts				
Poor relationships with patients				
Complaints				
Poor relationships between staff				
Disloyalty				
Accidents				
Poor decision making				

Continued

EXERCISE 6   Continued.

The study of GPs and practice managers found that they described the same six top effects of stress for staff, with slight differences in ranking of significance. How does your ranking compare with theirs?

Please complete the third column to show how your answers compared with the published reports of other GPs and practice managers. Rank your top six; add any of your top effects of stress at the bottom of the table in the 'Other' rows to display your top six. If you are different from the average GP or practice manager think why that is. Is it because you are unaware of certain effects of stress or are your circumstances different?

Effects of stress	GPs' rank order	Practice managers' rank order	Your rank order
Mistakes	1	1	
Arguments or angry outbursts	2	2	
Poor relationships with patients	3	4	
Poor relationships with staff	4	3	
Increased staff sickness	5	5	
Increased turnover	6	6	
Other:			
Other:			
Other:			
Other:			
Other:			

EXERCISE 7   Summarising sources and effects of stress for you.

This exercise will pull together all the work you have done throughout the module. By now you should have a good appreciation of the factors about you, your work, your home situation and life in general that are causing you stress. In this exercise look back at the answers you gave in the first five exercises and summarise the key causes of stress for you in each of the six categories, with respect to how you function at work and how you are outside work. The outcomes will include the result of the symptoms of stress on you or your organisation, for example 'mistakes' or 'rows at home'.

Sources of stress at work	Symptoms of stress (your own and organisational symptoms)	Outcomes
To do with the job itself		
Your role in the practice		
Your relationships at work		
Your career development		
Conflict at your home–work interface		
The practice organisation		
The NHS organisation		
Sources of stress outside work		
To do with your family/home		
Your role at home		
Your relationships with others outside work		
Your career development		
Conflict at your home–work interface		
The community or environment		

EXERCISE 8   Are you experiencing too much stress? Do you need help?

- Are you experiencing too much stress? Are you determined to act to minimise stress?

- Can you minimise the stresses in your life by yourself or do you need help?

Look back at Exercise 3. If a main cause for you is 'patient demands' and/or 'too much work' then you should go on to Module 2: Controlling stress in primary care, Module 3: Encouraging assertiveness skills and Module 4: Defining time management.

If a main cause for you is 'patient abuse or aggression' then you should go on to Module 3: Encouraging assertiveness skills, which also includes material on combating aggression.

If a main cause for you is 'the limited availability of appointments' you need to look at the practice organisation and controlling patient demand by working through Module 2: Controlling stress in primary care and Module 4: Defining time management.

If a main cause of stress for you is 'GP demands' you should work through Module 2: Controlling stress in primary care, Module 3: Encouraging assertiveness skills and Module 5: Enhancing job satisfaction.

If a main cause of stress for you is 'poor communication' you should go to Module 2: Controlling stress in primary care, Module 5: Enhancing job satisfaction and Module 6: Promoting career development to look at other opportunities.

Meantime what changes can you make:

- Today (name one)?

- Tomorrow (name two, however trivial)?

- Next week (name three, however small)?

References

1 Richards C (1989) *The health of doctors*. King's Fund, London.

2 Chambers R, George V, McNeill A, Campbell I (1998) Health at work in the general practice. *Br J Gen Pract.* **48**: 1501–4.

3 Howie J, Porter A, Heaney D, Hopton J (1991) Long to short consultation ratio: a proxy measure of quality of care for general practice. *Br J Gen Pract.* **41**: 48–54.

4 Chambers R, Campbell I (1996) Gender differences in general practices at work. *Br J Gen Pract.* **46**: 291–3.

5 Cox T (1993) *Stress research and stress management: putting theory to work*. HSE Contract Research Report No 61/1993. Health and Safety Executive, Suffolk.

6 Caplan RP (1994) Stress, anxiety and depression in hospital consultants, general practitioners and senior health service managers. *BMJ.* **309**: 1261–3.

7 Chambers R, Campbell I (1996) Anxiety and depression in general practitioners: associations with type of practice, fundholding, gender and other personal characteristics. *Fam Pract.* **13**(2): 170–3.

Other reading

Arroba T, James K (1992) *Pressure at work: a survival guide for managers*. McGraw-Hill Book Company, London.

Burnard P (1991) *Coping with stress in the health professions*. Chapman and Hall, London.

Haslam D (ed) (1994) *Not another guide to stress in general practice*. Medical Action Communications, UK.

Patel C (1991) *The complete guide to stress management*. Optima, London.

Woodham A (1995) *Beating stress at work*. Health Education Authority, London.

Video and relaxation tapes

Videos for Patients Ltd. For videos such as 'Stress': 122 Holland Park Avenue, London W11 4UA. Tel: 0171 229 5161; Fax: 0171 221 3832.

Wendy Lloyd Audio Productions Ltd. For audio cassette tapes such as the twin tapes of 'Coping with stress at work', 'The relaxation kit' and 'Feeling good': 30 Guffitts Rake, Meols, Wirral L47 7AD. Tel: 0151 632 0662.

MODULE 2
Controlling stress in primary care

AIMS

The aims of Module 2 are:

1 To increase GPs' understanding of the range of options and solutions that are likely to control or minimise stress.

2 To actively engage GPs in reducing a major source of stress.

3 To encourage GPs to make a timetabled action plan to reduce the stress in their lives.

4 To help GPs reduce the effects of their stress on their partner and/or family at home, and their GP partners and other members of the practice team at work.

CONTENTS

The total time to work through the module depends on the amount of time the reader spends reflecting on how the information in the module applies to him or her, before completing the exercises. The total time for which postgraduate education accreditation might be sought is nine hours (including time for reading and thinking and so long as the significant event analyses, stress reduction exercise and timetabled action plans are completed).*

---

* GP participants could apply to their region's Director of Postgraduate General Practice Education for permission to submit one or more completed modules for postgraduate education accreditation. Approval of such an application will be at the Director's discretion and may require the support of a local GP tutor in arranging assessment. No assessment will be undertaken by the author or Radcliffe Medical Press.

Here's what some GP participants said they had gained from undertaking the first *Survival Skills for GPs* programme:

'The course has helped to improve my confidence. It has been extremely beneficial to know that others have similar experiences and anxieties.'

'I felt a very different person when I started this module – I think I was actually quite dangerously stressed but now I feel more in control.'

'I feel reassured that I'm in the normal range of colleagues.'

'As a result (of doing the first module) I've already made several changes in the last few months to ease my stress.'

'The best part was realising that the feelings I have are those of stress, not a serious illness, and I can work through this.'

'I thought you might like to know what effect the stress management course had. I did take quite a long hard look at both work and personal stress. I decided I was overcommitted and reduced non-essential work drastically (e.g. I used to do six to seven DSS medicals per week; I reduced this to two, deciding it was pointless having the money but not the energy or time to enjoy it). I reorganised my surgery times so that they were realistic and I no longer had to "chase myself" because I was running late. I bought a coffee machine for my surgery (I know coffee is a potential stressor but it helps me). There were several other small (but cumulative) changes at work as well. I also joined a leisure club where there are trainers who monitor my progress in the gym (essential for me – to ensure regular attendance) and part of the programme involves relaxation at the end of training. I can take the family there as well. All told, I think the course had a big impact. I do feel much less pressurised. I still get the odd stress-filled day, but changes I have made make it easier to manage.'

'(The course) helped me look at myself and how I contribute to stresses and how I work towards stopping this.'

'I enjoyed being made to address my problems and identify ways of reducing my stress levels – for example, I would never have thought of changing my surgery arrangements without this stimulus.'

'...being made to think what I might do to help myself feel more in control rather than defeated all the time.'

'The programme forced me to look at what I do and the stress it induces and suggested/reinforced that I can change things.'

'It has taught me things about recognising and coping with stress that I did not know before.'

'Advice is also useful in helping stressed patients.'

'I enjoyed ... (the programme) ... it made me feel hopeful and enthusiastic that I can have some control of the situation.'

REDUCING STRESS EFFECTIVELY: OPTIONS AND SOLUTIONS

There are three types of responses to stress: physiological, psychological and behavioural reactions. The way you respond depends on personal factors such as age, gender, personality, previous family and personal experiences, as well as coping ability and other organisational options.

On the whole, many GPs do not think out plans to cope with the stresses in their lives and just hope for the best, often preferring avoidance and evasion techniques! Often, their struggles to overcome stress and reluctance to admit they are unable to cope mean that the stress problem becomes even worse.

Surveys of other primary care staff have shown that they do not tackle stresses systematically either, and put up with the stresses heaped upon them by their GPs in an unassertive way.

The kind of practical methods some GPs use to cope with stress at work are:

• seeking support from GP partners or family/friends

• sharing of problems with professional colleagues

• adoption of better time management practices

• more appropriate booking times for patients

• increased protected time off duty

• admission of doubts and worries to others

• achieving a better balance between work and home commitments.

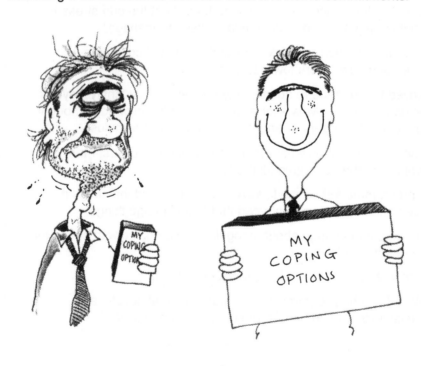

▼

Options and solutions.

It is difficult to make plans to cope with stress more effectively until you understand how you and others around you actually respond to stress. So the next section will explore your own responses to stress at work and home.

Having identified your main causes of stress you need to make a priority list. Some will require other members of the practice team to co-operate with a redistribution of tasks. Changes will have to be negotiated, especially if they involve amending other people's job descriptions after delegating some of your work to them. Such a reorganisation often benefits the whole practice if handled sensitively. Having delegated as many of your causes of stress as are practicable, you can still expect to retain a hard core with which you are stuck. To overcome or reduce these you will have to devise some strategies for coping with them.

First, you need to learn not to feel guilty. Ideal medical practice at all times is not possible and principles of good practice have sometimes to be sacrificed for expediency. So, tell yourself 'we're all human and make mistakes'.

Learn to relax so that you can make the most of any free period, even a few minutes. Try and train yourself to shut right off from your surroundings. You'll need a quiet room with no disturbances at the surgery or home, or even your car. Stop being a perfectionist and accept being 'good enough'. Adopting positive thinking and finding time for personal and professional development are vital. Have you considered whether you are setting your personal standards too high and aiming for excellence too much of the time?

There is a narrow line between behaving in an assertive or an aggressive, bossy way – sometimes it takes practice to get it right.

Avoid the seven deadly sins of the workaholic:

1 Stop being a perfectionist.

2 Don't judge your mistakes too harshly.

3 Resist the desire to control everything.

4 Learn to assertively decline extra commitments if you are already pressed for time.

5 Look after personal health and fitness.

6 Allow time for personal growth, the family and leisure.

7 Don't be too proud to ask for help.

The push for peak performance day after day can lead to burnout, whereas a sensibly planned programme, including protected time, can lead to optimal performance and a more balanced way of life. Let go a bit.

As well as lowering your standards to realistic levels, try reviewing to what degree you are in control of your own life at work and home and how much you need to be. Stop banging your head against a brick wall trying to control things you have no chance of changing. Become more laid back and reserve energy for being in control of things that really matter.

Stress can be either positive or negative, depending on how you perceive it and how you react to it. If you view new regulations as challenges, you will probably find ways of managing changes to your advantage, with

---

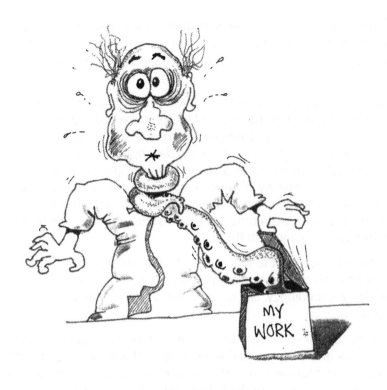

▼

Control over your work?

opportunities for learning and growth. Too many extra demands are impossible to absorb as opportunities and you must continually reassess your priorities.

Look after your health. Doctors tend to deny their own needs for rest and recuperation, feeling they are indispensable and playing down their own symptoms of illness. Compare how you behave when you are ill with what most people would do and try to narrow the gap.

Reduce outside commitments. Be sure of your motives for taking on commitments over and above your GP post. If you have just drifted into committee work or felt initially you couldn't say 'no', this might be the time for you to weigh up whether outside commitments are still worthwhile.

The objective of learning to cope better is to regain a balance between work and the rest of your life. One of the best coping methods of all, therefore, is not to take on the additional task or responsibility in the first place if it is not necessary. Just because you could do something well or find it interesting, or you are flattered to be asked, does not mean you should take it on when you are already pressed for time or distracted by other pressures.

This may require you to learn assertiveness skills and practise them at every opportunity. Assertiveness is about knowing and practising your rights – to change your mind, to make mistakes, to not understand about something (for example, the complex usages of the computer), to refuse demands, to express emotions, to be yourself without having to act for other people's benefit and to make decisions or statements without having always to justify them.

Be prepared to ask for help. Seeking support is a coping skill not often employed by GPs, who feel that it may be regarded as a sign of weakness or ignorance. Support networks may be used for another professional opinion, such as between practice staff or for emotional assistance. Encouraging GP partners and other members of the practice team to trust each other over sensitive issues may help defuse personal worries and stresses enormously. The support from others at the practice needs to be non-judgemental and a culture needs to be developed where people do not feel embarrassed or silly to be asking for help. GPs in a group partnership can feel lonely and isolated from colleagues, and fit into a macho culture where they are expected to keep their anxieties and stresses to themselves rather than burden their partners.

If a GP is fortunate enough to have a close and supportive spouse and family at home, that can be a good safe place to offload and share worries about work, so long as that does not stress relationships. Obtaining support from spouses or friends at home is just as important, if not more so. But it may not always be available as doctors are known for their high incidence of marriage breakdown and often have few friends outside work due to their workaholism and medicine-centred interests.

Much of this stiff-upper-lip veneer is learnt at medical school and can be cast off with practice. Who else will understand your worries about patients' complaints or excessive demands better than your work colleagues? If you express your feelings they may state theirs too, and together maybe you can do something about it.

Singlehanded GPs may have to look for support from other singlehanders by setting up a peer support group. But a better alternative may be to confide in one or more trusted members of the practice team, or a colleague from another practice. To stay fit and healthy involves physical, mental and spiritual well being.

To stay on top, you may need to regain your enthusiasm for learning and your quest for knowledge and understanding. The personal satisfaction from completing a project, degree course or some other educational experience is likely to make any GP more fulfilled and to reawaken an interest in all aspects of the practice.

Remember, it is not stress itself that is the damaging factor but your inability to cope with it. In a changing world you need to learn new ways of coping. That way lies survival.

GPs are vulnerable to stress because so many of their patients are anxious and stressed at coming to the doctor and fearful about their complaints. This anxiety, stress and fear can, unfortunately, be transferred to the doctors and staff they are consulting, causing a build up for them unless the doctors and staff are 'stress-proofed' or know how to reduce their own stress levels by developing their own personal strategies.

Don't forget – research into stress has shown that people with the best social supports who interact well with other people have the best ability to cope with stress, and are the least affected by it.

RESPONSES TO STRESS

EXERCISE 1   With whom do you discuss your troubles?

The list below gives various people with whom a GP might discuss ideas for coping with stress or seek help and advice. Put a tick in the column to indicate if you have ever sought advice or discussed ideas for coping with workload, stress or the demands from work. Tick if you have ever considered seeking advice or discussion on these topics with anyone listed. If there are people whom you could have approached but haven't, what has held you back?

	Have you sought advice or help or discussion?	*Would like to have sought advice, help or discussion*
Friend(s)		
Partners at work		
Spouse/partner or family member		
Other colleagues at work		
Own GP		
Occupational health staff		
Community psychiatric nurse		
Counsellor		
Mentor		
Practice/other manager		
Clergy		
Educationalist, e.g. GP tutor		
Skills course organiser		
Other:		

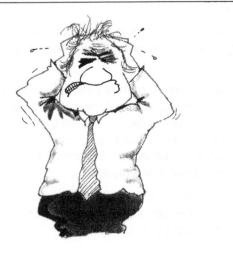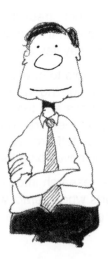

▼

Responses to stress.

EXERCISE 2   How do you usually respond to stress?

To reflect on how you usually respond to stress, complete the questionnaire below describing different types of response. The responses listed below are not ranked in any order of priority or markers of success. They have been identified by a group of young GPs as ways in which they cope with stress.[1] Please score each factor according to how you believe you usually respond (or n/a if it is not appropriate for you, e.g. you do not drive a car for 'driving at high speed'). If you often react with other types of responses that do not appear in the table, please add them to the bottom of the list. Last, rank in order of frequency the type of response you adopt most often.

Response to stress	Never or seldom	Sometimes	Often	Ranking
Seek discussion with colleagues or friends				
Drive at high speed				
Overeat				
Delegate tasks to practice staff				
Passive relaxation, e.g. TV, relaxation tape				
Have a complete break when not on duty				
Seek counselling				
Be irritable with colleagues or patients				
Drink more alcohol				
Take more exercise				
Manage time better				
Avoid stressful situations				
Feel anger towards patients or colleagues				
Use laughter or jokes				
Other:				
Other:				

Other responses might be to reduce caffeine/coffee, play music, get a pet, take up a new hobby, sleep, pray, yoga.

Compare your answers with the young GPs' range of responses.

Continued

EXERCISE 2 Continued.

GPs' ranking of types of responses to stress at work.

Response to stress	Ranking
Take a complete break	1
Seek discussion with colleagues or friends	2
Passive relaxation	3
Use laughter or jokes	4
Take more exercise	5
Feel anger towards patients or colleagues	6
Avoid stressful situations	7
Drink more alcohol	8
Manage time better	9
Overeat	10
Drive fast	11
Be irritable	12
Delegate tasks	13
Seek counselling	14

How similar was your ranking of your usual responses compared with these GPs? There were six 'good' responses in their top 10, but the other four types of response were all the kind which might make the circumstances worse, such as drinking more alcohol.

EXERCISE 3   How successful were the work-based coping methods you have tried in the past?

Please tick the column above to indicate which self-help action you have tried in the past. Was your response/action successful? Which of the methods described have you tried in the past? Note down briefly how you carried out the coping method, e.g. if you restricted paperwork – how, when and what? Do you still use that coping method? Did the coping method work for you and reduce your stress?

Coping method	Tried in the past? Yes/No	Was it successful? Yes/Partly/No
Reduce interruptions		
Decrease workload		
Restrict paperwork		
Plan for extra patients		
Better timed consultations		
Surgery more comfortable		
Limit doctor–patient relationship		
Others not mentioned:		

It is worth noting that one of the membership benefits of belonging to the BMA is the 'Supporters Scheme' that they run. If you are facing serious problems at work, your local office can introduce you to another doctor who will give you support and friendship to help you cope with emotional traumas. The volunteer supporters are trained. The BMA will also help in partnership disputes by offering advice and conciliating or mediating between both parties.

ACTING TO REDUCE STRESS AT WORK

Now that you have read through the synopsis of how GPs cope with stress and compared your own responses with how other doctors react to stress, you should have reflected on whether you've been adopting sensible coping methods or just letting things drift along. Read through the practical steps and tips on a range of coping methods that follows and then review how you have behaved in the past.

Surveys of stress in general practice uncover a long list of causes: interruptions, workload, paperwork, heartsink patients, patients' demands, complaints and so on. To minimise stress you first need to identify the prime causes as in Module 1 of this workbook and then make changes to reduce or avoid them.

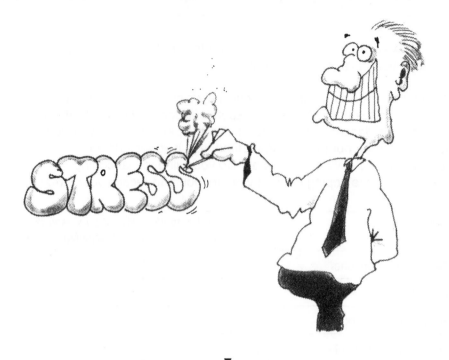

▼

Acting to reduce stress.

Reduce interruptions

People are stressed by situations over which they have little control, such as interruptions. If you go into the practice early to do paperwork, you will get little done and feel increasingly irritated if there are incessant telephone or staff enquiries.

- Restrict interruptions at designated times to clear your paperwork. Ask staff to stall enquiries until you are available.

- Unless you are the duty doctor, telephone interruptions during surgery times can be reduced to the number you choose to take.

- Change your system to suit you better – but obviously you must be accessible sometimes.

- Introduce a time when you are available for non-urgent requests.

Decrease workload

More work is being shifted from secondary care to primary care and patients are becoming more demanding. Your workload is therefore bound to increase unless you do something about it.

- Consider whether the practice can afford to appoint an extra partner or ancillary staff.

- Decide whether any of the practice work involved in home visiting, such as elderly checks, ear syringing or blood tests, can be diverted to district nurses or health visitors, or discontinued altogether.

- See what clinical work could be taken over by practice nurses. This might mean recruiting more nurses, extending their training or delegating some of their workload, such as paperwork, to ancillary staff.

- Reappraise whether you have the right balance between the amount of time you take off work and your earnings. Consider dropping inessential outside sessions if you are finding your workload too much, and managing on less money.

Restrict paperwork

Never complete routine paperwork that can be delegated to support staff.

- Sign claim forms and so on, but do not fill in any other details – leave it to others.

- Carry a tape recorder with you and dictate requests for staff to complete tasks for you.

- Complete the most complicated forms first when you are fresh.

- Never handle a letter or report more than once – read and act on it. If you procrastinate you will waste time rereading it later.

Plan for urgent, extra patients

One of the most stressful parts of conducting surgeries is the number of unexpected, extra patients added on at the end. This is best tackled as a practice.

- Everyone will need to agree a common policy and stick to it.

- There will have to be enough free slots to book same-day appointments for patients who have urgent problems requiring to be seen.

- Use the practice nurse as a triage nurse, once suitably trained, to reduce the number of extra patients booked with the GPs. Those having trivial problems might be assessed and dealt with more appropriately by a practice nurse.

- Whatever changes you decide on, the receptionists will be the linchpin in making the new system work, so involve them in your plans and welcome their suggestions – they may be too shy to suggest great ideas for improvements unless asked to help.

Time yourself

Time your consultations sensibly. If keeping to time is difficult and a major stress for you, consider altering the rate at which you book patients. If you always end your surgery 30 minutes late:

- book longer time slots

- discuss the possibility of the GPs all having different consultation times depending on the types of patients they attract and the GPs' various styles.

Make your surgery comfortable

- Review your consulting room and see how you can make it more comfortable or easier for you to work in.

- Rearrange your desk and the chairs, swop your chair if it makes your back ache, buy another storage cabinet if you want to tidy some of the papers away from view.

- Try a new position for the computer so that it's more accessible, and obtain a better display rack for referral and investigation forms.

- Treat yourself to some little item of luxury that will cheer you up on a bad day – a coffee maker for your own surgery, a new picture for your wall or a transistor radio to keep in your surgery for when you are doing paperwork.

Use visual distraction

- Make sure that there is something visual that is easily seen from your consulting room or reception chair that can be used to distract you when the going gets tough.

- A photograph of the family is the traditional answer but this may cause more problems than it's worth when patients persistently wish to chat about the members of your family appearing in the photograph, or your children object to their appearance several years on.

- Perhaps a holiday memento that you associate with happy times could be one of the best methods of transporting you from the stresses of practice life and remind you of the next holiday on your horizon.

Limit the intensity of your relationships with patients

Every GP knows that the closer the doctor–patient relationship is, the more it drains the GP. Obviously, if you never interact with your patients and 'give yourself' in any way, your work would be dissatisfying and that could be a source of stress in itself. But the converse is true and GPs should guard against becoming too involved with their patients' problems and emotions. Otherwise, they will find that their own family life will suffer as they become emotionally drained with too little energy and feelings left to give and exchange with their own partner and family.

- General practice work can too easily be all-consuming and take priority in GPs' own lives.

- It is difficult to maintain a distance in consultations with vulnerable patients whom the GP knows well and who have terrific problems with which the doctor sympathises. But somehow they have got to learn to maintain that distance and not be sucked into a whirlpool of human emotions and end up devoid of all feeling and burnt out themselves.

Easing the stress on a GP's family life

No family is immune from the pressures of modern life, and medical families have all the ingredients for fallout and breakdown. This is not to say you should be downhearted, but this is not an issue that should be swept under the carpet. The consequences of the pressures on GPs' families won't go away by wishful thinking and neglect. The pressures need to be examined and somehow faced, and if possible overcome.

Help is available though not always accepted, and there are common and recurring themes and pitfalls from which we can all learn, and solutions that others have found successful.

Communication

Whatever the causes, if tensions within the family are getting out of hand the priority is to re-establish better communication. The first step may be to try to distance yourself from your feelings about the situation and look from a different viewpoint.

Whole family approach: it sometimes helps to call a family meeting and let everyone have a chance to air their grievances or offer their ideas. Family members need to feel safe enough to speak honestly. But don't have too high expectations at first – they may need time and space to express themselves. This is not a 10 minute consultation, and it is important to get out of the doctor role and become an ordinary family member with good listening skills.

Sharing with your partner: another tack is to try and inject some freshness into your relationship with your partner. Make a date as in the old days and try to arrange regular outings for shared activities or interests. Acknowledge any problems with your sex life, if they exist. These are usually due to communication difficulties or lack of time alone together. If you make it a priority and show a little patience you will probably find some fun and laughter bubbling to the surface – a good sign.

Enjoying your children: try to arrange times when your children have your full attention. Talk about your work with them so they can be more understanding about your being away from home so much. Try to take more interest in what the children are up to and give more praise when you can. That means overcoming any tendency you might have to praise only academic or sporting success.

Family priorities: it is important to regularly re-evaluate those extra commitments that are keeping you away from the family, especially in the evenings and at weekends, and see if there are any you might drop. Do not see this as self-sacrifice, but as something you are doing as part of looking after yourself and your family. Get work-related worries off your chest when you come home and put them aside. Try and reduce work-related pressures on family life by, for example, not taking paperwork home. Perhaps employ caterers for your next work party, rather than expect colleagues and spouses to provide the supper.

Take time out: take regular holidays, and if you and your partners cover each other for holidays and courses, try to persuade your partners to employ a locum. The improved quality of life may justify the expense – ask the family!

Increase the efficiency of your practice organisation

If you are to function in as stress-free a way as possible then you will need to have an efficient and effective practice organisation behind you. That means overhauling the practice operation and making sure that the organisation is well managed. You and your staff should be well versed in modern theories of management, and communication should be well developed and regarded as being of high priority within the practice and within the PCG. Time and money should be invested in practice team development.

Stress reduction should be tackled by the whole team through dedicated courses and discussions/action plans amongst practice team members. All staff should know their 'rights' and what is expected of them. Practice procedures should be made explicit to staff and patients to minimise any misunderstandings. Complaints policies should be well advertised to practice staff and patients with the practice manager taking the lead with GP partners' backup whenever possible. Delegation should be optimised as far as resources and skills allow.

Continuing medical education offers one of the best ways to offset the stresses of modern general practice life, not only by providing a forum for discussion and mutual exchange of worries and solutions, but also by encouraging a life-long philosophy of professional development to cushion the practice staff against boredom and dissatisfaction with the daily grind.

Relaxation for stress relief

You have to find the method that works best for you. Some people find hard exercise more beneficial than deep relaxation. Why not buy or borrow a relaxation tape and see if it is helpful for you? Please do not listen to the tape whilst driving the car in case it makes you sleepy and less alert than usual. Choose a time and place when you are unlikely to be disturbed, lie back in an armchair or stretch out on a comfortable settee or bed, and play the tape through twice.

This may seem an easy part of the stress management module, but it is not. If you are someone who finds it difficult to relax, who becomes fidgety if they are waiting around with nothing to do, you will find that you have to be very firm with yourself to listen quietly to the relaxation sessions.

Different kinds of relaxation:

- short relaxation
- relax on the move
- step by step
- mental imagery.

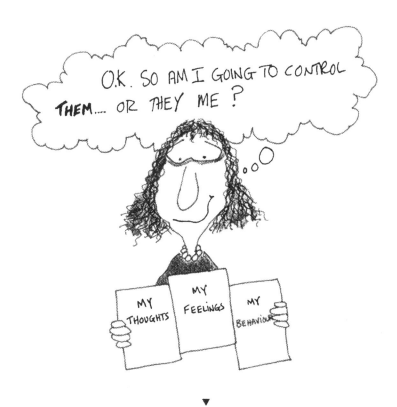

Thoughts + behaviour = stress.

EXERCISE 4   Where do you want to be? What will you do?

Write down below what actions/forms of self-help you intend to carry out in the near future to control stress. When will you start to do it?

Proposed self-help action	Start date
1	
2	
3	
4	
5	
6	

UNDERTAKE A SIGNIFICANT EVENT ANALYSIS OF STRESSFUL EVENTS

Next time you have an unusually stressful day at work or there is a critical situation where stress was the trigger factor or result, sit down to reflect and analyse what were the causes and consequences of the stress. Repeat the exercise for an extremely stressful event occurring outside work.

Analyse a significant event at work

STAGE 1: Write down a factual account of the stressful situation you have chosen – who was involved, what time of day, what task/activity you were doing.

For example, Dr Smith lost his temper after morning surgery and stormed into the reception area, shouting at the receptionists because 10 unexpected, extra patients had been added on to his list. That had made him late for his next appointment at a case conference meeting he'd really wanted to attend. So, those involved would be Dr Smith, the receptionists and the patients who overheard the row.

STAGE 2: Deduce the reasons for the crisis or stressful situation arising for your own case.

In this example, these were disorganised booking of appointments, with insufficient capacity for 'extras', and poor communication. Dr Smith had not informed the practice manager of his prior commitment.

STAGE 3: Record the effects of stress on the participants in the crisis or stressful situation you have chosen.

In the example here, Dr Smith was even later and left for the case conference feeling overwhelmingly angry and guilty and had difficulty concentrating once there. The practice manager and other staff took sides with the receptionists Dr Smith had shouted at, and were very aggrieved that Dr Smith had been so unfair. The receptionists Dr Smith had shouted at felt humiliated in front of the watching, waiting patients.

STAGE 4: Write down how you or others might have behaved differently, or how the practice organisation might be changed to reduce or eliminate the cause of stress you have nominated, from occurring.

In this instance, Dr Smith could have told the practice manager about his wish to attend the case conference as soon as he knew about it. The practice booking arrangements should be changed to allow sufficient spare capacity for extras. Dr Smith should agree to discuss any organisational problems or concerns with the practice manager in a private room.

Analyse a significant event outside work

STAGE 1: Write down a factual account of the stressful situation you have chosen – who was involved, the time of day, and the task/activity you or others were doing.

For example, Dr Smith came home far later than he had promised to find his wife in tears and his children had already left with a friend's parent for the school play they were acting in.

STAGE 2: Write down the reasons for the crisis or stressful situation arising from your specific situation.

In this example, Dr Smith was late because the surgery had ended later than he had hoped, his last three patients being the kind he classified as 'heartsink' patients. Then he was later still when one of the receptionists had asked him to sort out problems with several repeat prescriptions and he'd had to call in on an old lady he'd told he'd revisit that week and hadn't had time to do earlier. But, to be honest, he had forgotten about the school play and that he had promised to be home in good time for it.

STAGE 3: Write down the effects of stress on the participants in the crisis or stressful situation you have chosen.

In this instance, Dr Smith's children thought he cared more about his work than them (and they were right!) and because it had happened to them so many times before they were cold-hearted about the situation and the bond with their father was weakened even further. Dr Smith's wife was upset, being torn between loyalty to her husband and respecting the importance of his job as a GP, and her duty as a mother; this was another stage in her increasing feelings of resentment towards her husband for putting his family last. Dr Smith was secretly glad he'd got out of going to the school play but dismayed to find he had to comfort his wife and show yet another human being some sympathy and kindness, just when he thought he'd left his patients behind and could turn that sort of behaviour off for the day.

STAGE 4: Record how you or others might have behaved differently, or how the practice/home organisation might be changed, to reduce or eliminate the cause of stress you have nominated from occurring.

In this instance, Dr Smith could have prioritised his family's needs and arranged to return home in plenty of time, leaving spare minutes for any unforeseen eventuality at work. He could have booked his surgery earlier, told the receptionists he'd sort out the repeat prescriptions in the morning and phoned the old lady he'd promised to revisit to explain he was postponing his call until tomorrow. The family need not make changes as they could rightfully expect Dr Smith's attendance at the school play.

EXERCISE 5   Now undertake your own significant event audit of stress at the practice, and another for a stressful event arising from outside work.

Analyse a significant event at work

STAGE 1: Write down a factual account of the stressful situation you have chosen – who was involved, the time of day, and the task/activity you or others were doing.

STAGE 2: Write down the reasons for the crisis or stressful situation arising from your specific situation.

STAGE 3: Write down the effects of stress on the participants in the crisis or stressful situation you have chosen.

STAGE 4: Record how you or others might have behaved differently or how the practice organisation might be changed to reduce or eliminate this cause of stress from occurring.

The plan for a significant event outside work

STAGE 1: Write down a factual account of the stressful situation you have chosen – who was involved, the time of day, and the task/activity you or others were doing.

STAGE 2: Write down the reasons for the crisis or stressful situation arising from your specific situation.

STAGE 3: Write down the effects of stress on the participants in the crisis or stressful situation you have chosen.

STAGE 4: Record how you or others might have behaved differently or how the practice/home organisation might be changed to reduce or eliminate the cause of stress you have nominated from occurring.

FINDING YOUR OWN SOLUTIONS

Only you can identify the best solutions for you! It may help to decide which stress-reducing interventions you want to make, to classify interventions as:

- preventive, that is reducing or changing the nature of the stressor, to remove the 'hazard' or reduce the frequency/extent of the stressor

- secondarily altering your individual response to stress or improving the practice's ability to recognise and deal with stress-related problems as they arise

- minimising the effects of stress, to heal/help those who have been traumatised or stressed by their work, or to help staff cope with and recover from problems at work.

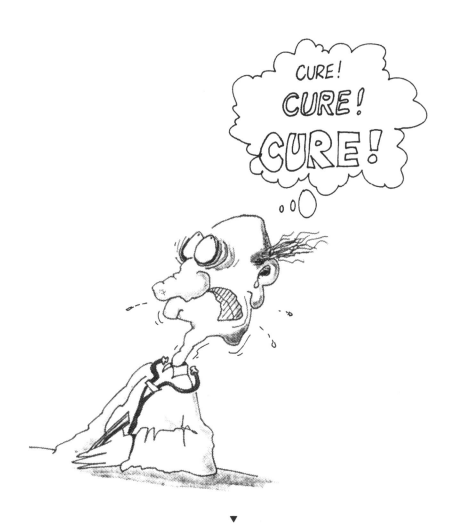

▼

Finding your own solutions.

EXERCISE 6   Finding your own solutions.

Will you reduce stress at a:

- practice organisational level?

- practice level to support the staff (including GPs)?

- personal level to improve the management of your work and reaction to stress?

STAGE 1: Choose which cause of stress you wish to tackle first, and whether you will tackle a primary, secondary or tertiary intervention for you as an individual or the practice organisation. This should be: a frequent source of stress; an important cause of stress; an infrequent stress that when it occurs has far-reaching effects; or a stress which is costly in terms of time or resources. It must be a realistic choice, i.e. a cause of stress which you can reasonably expect to be able to reduce.

STAGE 2: Set a 'standard' (agreed with others from the practice/or from published literature/or pick a sensible target to aim at), i.e. a goal that is a recognisable measurement of an acceptable lower level of the stress you hope to achieve after you have introduced a new system to reduce the cause of that stress.

You may need to carry out baseline data collection first to provide sufficient information to set the standard if there is no obvious reference point. Standards might be agreed levels of personal well being, time measurements, amount of work delegated, new system(s) in practice procedures, extent of communication in the practice, etc.

STAGE 3: Write out a plan to reduce the stress, including the expected outcomes and the expected benefits and disadvantages. Discuss your proposal with everyone else involved, at home and at work. Obtain the agreement of anyone who may be concerned by the proposed changes to your set standard(s) and your proposed intervention(s). Amend your plans in the light of others' comments. This stage will include obtaining or buying any extra equipment, training yourself or others if new skills are required, applying for extra staff time or making other resource or organisational arrangements.

STAGE 4: Record current performance as a baseline before making any changes.

STAGE 5: Introduce and carry out intervention. Record new performance measures.

Continued

EXERCISE 6 Continued.

STAGE 6: Compare the new performance with the old performance, and with pre-set standards. Has the agreed standard been reached? Feed back information about comparison of performance, outcomes of intervention(s) and the improvements or changes to those involved in, or affected by, the project. Agree and make further changes if standards were still not met. Arrange further training, etc., if current skills still inadequate.

STAGE 7: Monitor performance, including your well being, three to six months later. Reinforce interventions and/or changes, etc., as necessary.

And finally

Armed with the knowledge of what seems to cause you the most stress at work and at home (from your daily stress logs in Module 1), and what the effects of those stressors are (from your completed questionnaires and own stress performance curve in Module 1 and the significant event audits in this Module), you are now in a position to think out plans to reduce the stresses in your life.

EXERCISE 7 Specify exactly what you intend to do, why, when and how. Choose three more key sources of stress for you and make plans to tackle them in the near future:

1

2

3

For each source use the following framework and make a timetabled action plan.

- What stress will you tackle?

- Why have you chosen this particular source of stress?

- What will you do?

- When will you do it?

- What other changes will you need to make or what resources will you need to buy?

- Will the changes involve altering how other people do things?

- What do you expect to be the outcome of your plan?

References

1 Chambers R, Wall D, Campbell I (1996) Stresses, coping mechanisms and job satisfaction in general practitioner registrars. *Br J Gen Pract.* **46**: 343–8.

Other reading

Arroba T, James K (1992) *Pressure at work: a survival guide for managers.* McGraw-Hill Book Company, London.

Burnard P (1991) *Coping with stress in the health professions.* Chapman and Hall, London.

Haslam D (ed) (1994) *Not another guide to stress in general practice.* Medical Action Communications, UK.

Patel C (1991) *The complete guide to stress management.* Optima, London.

Woodham A (1995) *Beating stress at work.* Health Education Authority, London.

Video and relaxation tapes

Videos for Patients Ltd. For videos such as 'Stress': 122 Holland Park Avenue, London W11 4UA. Tel: 0171 229 5161; Fax: 0171 221 3832.

Wendy Lloyd Audio Productions Ltd. For audio cassette tapes such as the twin tapes of 'Coping with stress at work', 'The relaxation kit' and 'Feeling good': 30 Guffitts Rake, Meols, Wirral L47 7AD. Tel: 0151 632 0662.

MODULE 3
Encouraging assertiveness skills

AIMS

The aims of Module 3 are:

1 To remind GPs of the advantages of assertive behaviour.

2 To encourage GPs to adopt assertive behaviour.

3 To engage readers in developing and practising assertiveness skills.

CONTENTS

The total time to work through the module depends on the amount of time the GP reader spends reflecting on how the information in the module applies to him or her, before completing the exercises. The total time for which postgraduate education accreditation might be sought is six hours, including time for reading and thinking and completing all the exercises.*

---

* GP participants could apply to their region's Director of Postgraduate General Practice Education for permission to submit one or more completed modules for postgraduate education accreditation. Approval of such an application will be at the Director's discretion and may require the support of a local GP tutor in arranging assessment. No assessment will be undertaken by the author or Radcliffe Medical Press.

Here's what some GP participants said they had gained from undertaking the first *Survival Skills for GPs* programme:

'I found the section on assertiveness and self-esteem particularly helpful.'

'I had to read/do all of it – hence look at some issues I find unpalatable.'

'It has given me insight and foundations for looking into and identifying my own stress.'

'The module has been much *better* than expected and made me realise that the feelings I have are felt by others too, but we don't admit it to each other.'

'What I liked is the idea one can have a handle on events and emotions.'

WHAT IS BEING ASSERTIVE ABOUT?

Being assertive is about expressing your feelings clearly and openly and behaving in keeping with these feelings in an honest way. Being assertive is not the same as being aggressive. It is about deciding what you want to do or to happen, judging if it's reasonable or not and acting accordingly.

A GP's natural instinct is to help people, and even those who are hopelessly overworked will often take on extra tasks when they know it's crazy to do so. Assertiveness in the work context is about you facing up to the fact that everybody has a limit to their time and energy, and politely but firmly refusing to take on extra work if you know it will cause you to be overstretched, or refusing to be manipulated by others.

Assertiveness is certainly not about getting what you want all the time. Nor is it about being a perfectionist and driving yourself and others into the ground. It's about being prepared to stick up for yourself if you think you're right whilst at the same time being willing to reach a compromise with others.

To be successful at being assertive you've got to understand the tricks others employ to get their own way. Some patients can be devious, dropping hints about what they really want but placing the onus on you to decide exactly what it is. This is ridiculous. You've got better things to do with your time and energies than play these sorts of games. Faced with this sort of patient, state clearly and simply what you think is the best and refuse to be side-tracked. If the patient tries to blackmail you, for example by saying 'well, you know best doctor, but I do hope I don't have to call you out later', stick to your guns.

If people try to bully you, and persist even after you've told them 'no', don't give in. Giving in just for some peace and quiet will make things a hundred times worse, and you will feel resentful as well as stressed. Keep saying calmly but firmly: 'I don't think you heard me, I'm not prepared to do that.' It's important to resist the temptation to get angry. Disarm the anger of a patient or colleague by acknowledging their feelings and staying calm. But don't give in.

Passive behaviour in others can be especially difficult to handle, as it is a technique health professionals fall for, not liking to seem to take advantage of someone when he/she's down. You are made to feel selfish if you ignore the 'victim's' wishes or hesitant requests. Be careful. You might end up doing what the passive person wants you to do rather than live with the guilt of pleasing yourself. Respond by stating specifically what you want with a simple explanation. When the next patient needles you, saying 'no-one cares anymore about people' or 'I expect it's all my fault', and you feel yourself tempted to reassure them to the contrary, think of the game they are playing. They are trying to manipulate you. Don't fall for it!

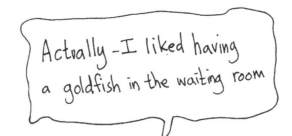

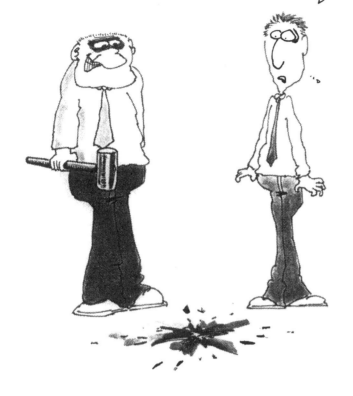

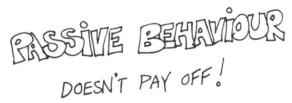

Being assertive.

One of the characteristics of someone who is healthily assertive is that they are not afraid to give their opinion. Nobody should be afraid to give their opinion on a subject they know something about.

And not only do you have as much right to be heard as anybody else, you also have the right to change your mind. If you decide that on reflection you don't want to take on a task, don't be afraid to say so.

The potential advantages for you of being assertive are:

- increased self-confidence

- increased control over your emotions

- people will relate to assertive people more readily than to those who are passive or aggressive
- increased self-respect
- people being more likely to respond with assertive behaviour as they don't feel threatened or browbeaten
- increased respect from others
- being more likely to achieve satisfactory changes.

How assertive are you now?

How do you generally behave at work:

- passively, just letting things happen to you without letting your feelings be known?
- assertively, stating clearly what you want and/or how you feel?
- being abrasive, aggressive or overbearing to order things how you want them to be, without regard or respect for other peoples' feelings and views?

EXERCISE 1   Reflect on how you usually behave and feel if…

1 One of the GPs has decreed that there will be no locum doctors booked whilst he and another doctor are away on holiday; the consequences are that patients are clamouring for appointments that don't exist, the other GPs and the practice nurses have extended surgeries finishing over an hour late, and the receptionists are taking flak from all sides. Do you think you would:

a Keep your head down, work harder than ever and say nothing, but seethe inside?

b Arrange an urgent conference with others in the practice to plan best ways of coping and feed back facts of situation to all the GPs so that the locum ban can be reconsidered?

c Bawl out anyone giving you extra work and vent your feelings on the absent GP's home answerphone?

2 It's 5.00 pm and you have everything planned out. There's another hour left of surgery, then you are off home for a leisurely bath before a trip to the theatre with your partner to see a play you have been really looking forward to. Suddenly your plans are dashed. A slip of paper is hurriedly thrust into your hands telling you to come to an urgent meeting after surgery, called by a local GP to discuss the Health Authority's new rules – your practice income might be threatened. Do you:

a Phone home apologetically and say you will be late and so will go straight from work, meeting your spouse/partner at the theatre?

Continued

---

b Explain to the perpetrator of the note that you recognise the reason for meeting is important, that you are willing to meet as soon as it is mutually convenient, but are unable to go to the meeting after surgery?

c Storm into the meeting after surgery has ended and disrupt it by broadcasting your views on the matter, forcing a quick decision and rushing home in an angry mood with no time to wash and change?

3 You are quietly getting on with practice paperwork whilst there is a lull between surgeries. Ellen comes to reception and asks for a prescription to take away. She is terribly apologetic, she knows she is a trouble to you and she shouldn't be bothering you with her problems when you are so busy, but she has just slipped out whilst her mother whom she cares for is asleep, and it would be great if she could have the prescription now. Do you:

a Just say nothing and do the prescription for her as that is the easiest option?

b Explain why the practice rules for requesting and receiving prescriptions have been made to safeguard the patients and maximise practice efficiency, slotting her request into the practice system?

c Gesture angrily to the notice about requesting prescriptions and tell her you are far too busy to deal with her request now?

Code: a = passive or unassertive, b = assertive, c = aggressive.

Was your response to these scenarios generally 'passive or unassertive', 'assertive' or 'aggressive'? These might seem extreme examples of each type of behaviour, but I expect you can recognise traits in yourself as being likely to mean that you usually behave passively or aggressively under these sort of conditions.

Non-verbal behaviour: the body language that gives you away

Passive	Assertive	Aggressive
Covers mouth with hand	Direct eye contact	Gesticulates expansively
Looks down at the floor	Head erect	Clenched/pounding fists
Constant shifting of weight	Descriptive hand gestures	Finger pointing
Fiddles with clothing or jewellery	Emphasises key words	Hands on hips
Rubs head or parts of body	Steady, firm voice	Rigid posture
Frequent nodding of head	Open movements	Strident voice
Throat clearing	Relaxed	Stares others down

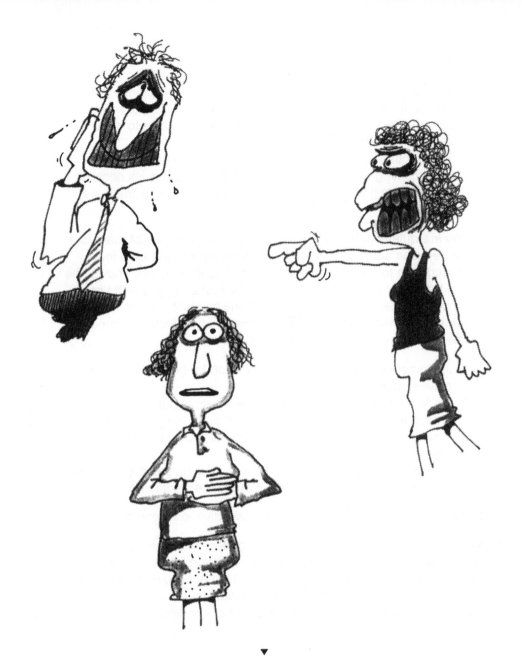

Passive / assertive / aggressive.

EXERCISE 2   Consider your usual body language when in situations where you disagree with others over an issue you consider to be important.

Do you recognise your non-verbal behaviour patterns from the list on the previous page as mainly 'passive', mainly 'assertive' or mainly 'aggressive' in a:

- situation at work with a patient?

- situation at work with fellow GPs?

- situation outside work with a shop assistant?

- situation outside work with a member of your family?

Are you consistent? Do you behave differently at work from how you do at home or in another community setting? Could you change your non-verbal behaviour and the signals you give out so that you are more consistent?

What can you do to be more consistently assertive

1 To be treated with respect

- Tell others what you want and need, what you like and don't like, express positives first and negatives second.

- Take pride in your appearance and believe in yourself.

2 To have and express feelings and opinions

- Use the 'broken record' technique, calmly repeating your original statement (at an appropriate time and place).

- Let others know what you are feeling; your vulnerability and trust in others will encourage them to confide in you too.

3 To be listened to and taken seriously

- Match your body language to your assertive message, i.e. stay calm and serious, avoid frivolous quips and use direct eye contact.

- Back up your proposals with well thought out reasons for changes.

- Initiate and get involved in conversations, don't wait for others to approach you first.

4 To set your own reasonable priorities

- Set your own goals; dismantle barriers to achieving your goals.

5 To say 'no' without feeling guilty

- Use simple, direct language.

- Deflect other people's attempts at distracting you from your purpose; acknowledge you have heard the other person's viewpoint and repeat your response.

- Distance yourself from problem situations until you get a handle on what's going on, and can be adequately prepared for a considered response.

- Do not lose self-control and become angry or ill-tempered.

6 **To choose not to assert yourself**

- Try 'active listening': listen, clarify, summarise and paraphrase a speaker's words to improve your understanding of their meaning.

7 **To view your needs as important as those of others**

- Learn to recognise the control tactics others are using and be ready to counter them: interrupt back, use flattery, engage them as advisers, ask for information if you are excluded from a conversation by cryptic remarks.

Transactional analysis

This is another technique to use to become more aware of your personality and style and how you relate to and communicate with others. This divides personality into three components: parent, adult and child. The child is the dependent part of your personality, that was the earliest part to develop. It consists of the 'free' child who feels, wants and needs emotion and creativity, and the 'adapted' child that has learnt how to fit in with other people through pleasing them, gaining approval and manipulation. The adult component is the rational, logical part of the personality that thinks objectively, works out problems and makes decisions. The parent part of the personality looks after the person, as the 'critical' parent issuing advice and judging shortcomings and the 'nurturing' parent who helps, supports and cares for themself.

Dealing with others adopting a child state will bring out the 'parent' in you and vice versa. The adult state is the one you should aim to adopt and expand as far as possible; adult to adult communication is the essence of assertiveness.

Tips for assertiveness

1 Say 'No' clearly and then move away or change the subject. Keep repeating 'No' – don't be diverted.

2 Be honest and direct with everyone.

3 Don't apologise or justify yourself more than is reasonable.

4 Offer a workable compromise and negotiate an agreement that suits you and the other party.

5 Pause before answering a 'Yes' you'll regret. Delay your response and give yourself more time to think by asking for more information.

6 Be aware of your body language and keep it as assertive as possible. Match your tone to your words (don't smile if you are giving a serious message).

7 Persistently repeat your message in a calm manner to someone who is trying to pressurise you to do something you don't want to do. Don't be side-tracked.

8 Show you are listening to the other person's point of view and giving them a fair hearing.

9 Practise expressing your opinion and rights rather than expecting other people to guess what you want.

10 Don't be too hard on yourself if you make a mistake – everyone is human.

11 Be confident enough to change your mind if that is appropriate.

12 It can be assertive to say nothing.

Keep practising assertiveness until it comes naturally. Other people are often unaware of their own behaviour and making an assertive response to an aggressive person may make them realise how they have been behaving. Be aware that if you are angry, it is unlikely you will manage to be assertive. Challenge people who are sulking and invite them to tell you if they have a problem. If they deny they have a problem treat them normally and don't mention the matter again.

EXERCISE 3   Working through the stages of assertiveness.

Think of an example of a situation at work that occurred in the last few days in which you behaved passively or aggressively, and wish you had been more assertive. Describe the situation:

Who was involved?

Where did the event happen?

What triggered the episode?

How did you behave? Were you pushy, shy, obnoxious, uncompromising?

How did the other person respond?

Continued

Encouraging assertiveness skills

EXERCISE 3 Continued.

How well did you communicate your feelings?

Did you handle any conflict well?

What was the outcome of the exchange?

What should you have done or said?

EXERCISE 4 What are your views on the appropriateness of being assertive with others at work and outside work?

Do you think that there are any disadvantages to being assertive?

Do you have any reservations about becoming more assertive?

List below the people at work or outside work with whom you intend to be more assertive now and what you expect the outcome(s) to be.

Intend to be more assertive with	Likely outcome(s)
1	
2	
3	
4	
5	

PROMOTE YOUR MESSAGE OR NEGOTIATE YOUR CAUSE ASSERTIVELY

This section gives some practical advice on using assertive behaviour to:

- promote a new message or cause

- negotiate new working conditions or the setting up of a new scheme.

Promote your message or cause assertively ...

...if you want to change the way your practice works, introduce a new initiative, persuade the Health Authority to support your ideas or influence primary care developments in the community, you will be most likely to succeed in promoting your message or cause by planning out every stage of your 'mini-campaign' and using an assertive approach. There will be plenty of opportunities in the near future, as primary care groups establish themselves, for getting your message across about a particular cause or way of working dear to your heart.

If you hector or bully work colleagues or external organisations such as the Health Authority into doing what you want, you might get superficial agreement to your plans and ideas, but you will not achieve their lasting commitment and successful change in the long run. Aggression does not pay off long term.

This section should provoke your thoughts on the lateral thinking and persistence required to put a new message across. You will develop your own individual perspective on how best you can influence change: everyone has their own style. Value yours.

Know yourself well

- Understand your own motivation for instigating the change and the extent of altruism *versus* self-promotion (be ready for critics).

- Know your strengths and weaknesses, your preferred style. Do you understand your own personality profile, are you extrovert/ introvert? Whichever it is, select mediums in which you are comfortable and perform well, such as committee meetings, networking with others, speaking on the local radio, one-to-one exchanges, presenting at local professionals' meetings.

- Decide if the message is important enough to be worth the effort. Your passion for the cause will have to motivate you for months/years. Your genuineness will show and help to sell your message.

- Be aware of your effect on people – then you can either deflect their criticisms or rationalise their support or hostility.

- Get into the way of thinking you can do anything if you want to do so enough. You don't need money to start, you are your own resource.

- Don't be a perfectionist, there's not time.

- Protect yourself from emotional overload – you will get 'sad' cases who try to latch on to your strength. Set your own boundaries and be assertive. Don't feel guilty that you cannot help everybody. If you choose a central organisational role to promote your message you cannot offer many individuals succour too.

- Remember everybody doesn't have to like you.

- Don't let adulation and meeting the 'nobs' (if either apply!) go to your head – you are still just you and a small cog in a mammoth wheel.

- Don't expect admiration, thanks or acknowledgement – there's a lot of jealousy, hostility and backbiting out there if you seem to be successful. Your self-worth and achievement of tasks set will have to keep you going. A few faithful colleagues/family are all that's needed, but they are vital.

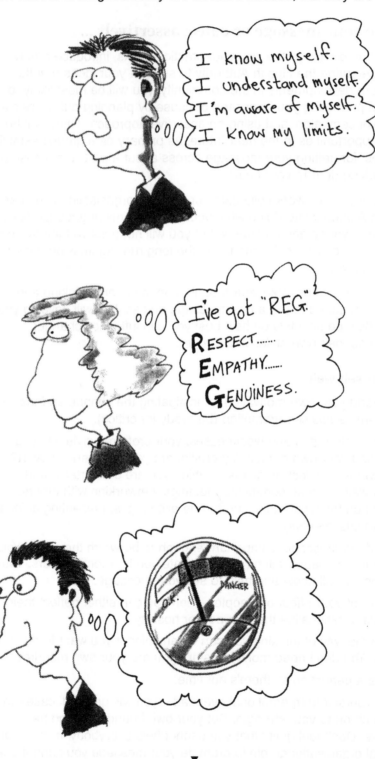

Know yourself.

Prepare well

- Prepare well for any meeting. Try to make sure your business is towards the top of the agenda (unless you want it nodded through when everyone is tired!). Circulate briefing papers before the meeting and have the answers ready to any queries that might arise, so that the meeting can agree an action plan and not postpone decision making until more information is available.

- Don't be caught out, whether it is a radio broadcast, local meeting or an enquiry in the corridor or street. Get training in skills you lack – writing, speaking, audiovisual aids, broadcasting.

- Do your homework well first, to develop your key message so it's on a sound and valid base, and you won't be taken unawares if new facts come to light.

- Find out the name of people at the top if writing letters.

- Keep good notes about people you contact, their activities, aspirations, plans for the future.

Deliver your message clearly

- Be consistent – same message, repetitive sound bites. Decide early on key words and messages; be faithful to your own style.

- Deliver your message as appropriate for your colleagues, audience or readership – right words (level and 'language'), in tune with their culture, showing how your cause or change will benefit them.

- Leave something about you or your message behind when you talk or meet people whenever possible, e.g. handouts or business cards, have some with you.

Deliver your message consistently

- Be persistent... follow people up... send them reminders of your work... again... and again...

- Don't waste effort. If you prepare a handout, use it for an article. Practise good time management, do tricky writing when fresh and keen.

- Don't duplicate others' work, build on it. Collaborate so long as you don't end up doing the work for others.

Deliver your message cleverly

- Tackle the promotion of your cause or message from different angles, or through different disciplines.

- Stay in touch and find continuing new material. Update your basic message and ways of promoting it or tangential issues (but not detracting from the basic message). Be creative and surprise people.

- Find ways to orchestrate a 'campaign' or momentum that uses others to promote your message. You will not have much influence as just one solitary voice.

- Find out who has the power/is important and work out ways to influence them. How do they think? What do they need? Can you supply it? Can you give them what they need without making enemies?

- Don't criticise people thoughtlessly. You might be wrong, so find out more. Your criticisms might alienate people who could help promote your message. On the other hand don't take any unjustified remarks lying down.

- Gather enough resources by hook or crook to have an assistant to support you, take messages, gatekeep, etc.

Accept credit where credit's due

- Never deny you are an 'expert' (who is?). Always accept other peoples' praise – it's only superficial anyway and they may be saying the opposite tomorrow. Don't be humble – they are lucky that you exhaust yourself promoting the cause and there probably is no-one else who knows more (even if that's too little in your own estimation).

- Don't let others take credit for what you have done – put your name on everything, send original copies to anyone senior who you think might not realise where the work has come from, attend all important functions you are invited to as far as your diary lets you.

Don't get too tired of your message – have other interests too – they will be likely to be 'up' when other issues/feedback is 'down'. Variety keeps you zingy.

How you promote your message depends on what it is, your circumstances and your own style. You have to find your own way, reflecting on progress as you go.

EXERCISE 5   Plan out how you might promote a new cause that others around you do not instantly embrace.

You want to set up a patient participation group in your practice. No-one has ever mooted such a move in your practice before. You don't know for sure, but you think the idea will be scorned when you first introduce it. How should you go about the challenge of establishing such a group? Map out brief answers to the following framework:

1 What is your motivation for setting up such a patient participation group?

2 Why should it be you who is involved?

Continued

EXERCISE 5 Continued.

3 How will you prepare for the challenge of setting up a patient participation group?

4 What will your key message be?

5 How and where will you deliver your message?

6 How will you influence other colleagues at work?

7 What is your action plan?

Example answers to the challenge of how to go about setting up a patient participation group:

• What is your motivation?

You believe in genuine participation of the patient population in planning and monitoring primary care in the practice. You would like to work in a leading practice. Such an initiative will fit in with the philosophy of NHS developments on engaging the public. It may save you work at no cost if members of a patient participation group give the practice practical help – by fundraising for equipment, doing chores for the housebound, organising a practice newsletter, etc.

• Why should it be you who is involved?

No-one else has the vision or commitment to organise such an initiative.

• How will you prepare for the challenge of setting up a patient participation group?

Find out what other practices have done – phone up the practice managers of any such groups elsewhere and find out what works well and what doesn't. Ask the Health Authority for help – any literature, experienced facilitator, resources.

• What is your message?

Think out the potential benefits to everyone in the practice – GPs, practice manager, staff, patients. Prepare your case accordingly, giving an honest appraisal of the advantages and drawbacks.

• How will you deliver your message?

Plan the preliminary information needed to seed your ideas around the practice. Follow usual procedures for introducing new ideas – put it on the agenda for the next staff or partnership meeting.

Continued

• What is your action plan?

A timetabled programme should include details of how to involve all concerned, information gathering and presentation until a decision has been made. A second action plan will be needed to implement the initiative, whilst consulting everyone on the shape of the new scheme, refining the details according to their input, being fair to everyone involved as far as possible.

Develop assertive negotiating skills

Negotiating is an integral part of assertive behaviour that is used to reach an agreement that is mutually acceptable to both sides.

Prepare your arguments well using logic based on facts and figures rather than offering veiled threats or empty promises. Give a fair assessment of the current situation, not exaggerating or minimising the problems, issues or challenges involved.

You will need to be clear about your objectives in any negotiations, however minor. If you are negotiating for others, you will need a clear brief from them to be sure that their objectives coincide with yours, and to know how far you are mandated to go on their behalf. You must not exceed their brief or you may find you have negotiated an unworkable new arrangement that others disclaim.

State your most important requirements clearly in a straightforward manner. Describe the benefits for the other party – if it is a new scheme at work it might be more clinically effective, more cost-effective or more convenient for GPs, staff or patients.

Listen carefully to the other person's viewpoint, and understand their position and concerns. Clarify what they are saying and their position and the exact terms and conditions they are offering. Summarise what you think they have just said to check out the wording and ensure that there are no ambiguities. Ask open questions to obtain information, and find out what their 'bottom line' is. Look for weaknesses or unfairness in their arguments.

Avoid confrontation or a stalemate by offering other options which you have worked out beforehand as being acceptable alternative solutions. Discuss how each party might trade concessions to reach an acceptable agreement; if the other person makes a concession don't crow. For the negotiations to remain amicable, it's important to both parties to avoid loss of face. Give the other person time to reflect on your request and work through your suggested ideas or changes, rather than demand an instant response.

Once agreement is reached, close the discussion. Ruminating back through the problems or different options will only be time-wasting and the other party may try and reopen negotiations or backtrack on your agreement.

EXERCISE 6   Practise negotiating over an issue you care about now.

Think of something you have been wanting to change at work that you have not yet discussed with the others. You should expect that the change will benefit you and not disadvantage others, although it may require them to work in a different way.

What is the change that you intend to negotiate (choose a minor issue for your first attempt)?

What are the potential advantages for you, and for others?

What are the potential disadvantages for you, and for others?

What facts relate to your case (the full facts, winners and losers)?

Who will the change affect, and how will they be affected?

How and where will you put your case?

What is your 'bottom line', i.e. what is the limit or extent of changes you propose that will satisfy your purpose?

What is likely to be the others' 'bottom line'?

Have you other ideas or suggestions to offer that might be used as bargaining tools?

What are your plans for tackling which people, when and where?

FEELING GOOD BY RAISING YOUR SELF-ESTEEM

We know from published research that doctors tend to have low self-esteem. Some people blame the traditional methods of training at medical school where students are often ridiculed by senior, trained staff for their ignorance, and where the culture of doctors' expected infallibility prevails. Then when the medical students graduate and find they cannot reach uniformly perfect standards and do actually make mistakes, self-esteem is lowered. High levels of self-criticism are strong predictors of doctors' feeling stressed so that raising your self-esteem and learning to tolerate failures in yourself are important targets to attain in your fight against stress.

Individuals can deliberately change their self-esteem by positive tactics and thinking. But to effect any change you have to be prepared to take the risk of failure – success is not automatic. And to ride failures successfully you have to develop a positive approach before you start so that you can set yourself up to learn from failure rather than be cast down by it.

Some positive strategies to raise your self-esteem are:

1 Accept that not every attempt to change will be a success.

2 Be prepared to take a risk to effect a change in your life.

3 Try positive visualisation, that is imagine yourself successfully managing a forthcoming event or activity about which you are feeling apprehensive.

4 Use positive body language – people will treat you more positively too.

5 Review and recall past successes and hold them in the forefront of your mind.

6 Learn from any mistakes or failures and don't dismiss such experiences.

7 Learn to feel comfortable with yourself – physically and mentally.

8 Write your worries down and review them periodically rather than continually fretting over them.

9 Be aware of your good points and constantly reinforce them in your thinking.

10 Do the best for yourself and give yourself every opportunity to succeed – don't set yourself up to fail.

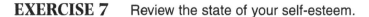

EXERCISE 7   Review the state of your self-esteem.

Do you need to concentrate on trying to raise your self-esteem?
If so, write down any positive strategies you could take to raise your
self-esteem. If your self-esteem is pretty good what can you do to
maintain it? What will you do and when?

1

2

3

4

When will you review the outcomes of this exercise?

AVOIDING AGGRESSION AND VIOLENCE IN GENERAL PRACTICE

The best way to reduce stress from aggression and violence is to prevent
the episode occurring in the first place. This will include:

- avoiding potentially dangerous situations especially on-call and on
  home visits
- learning how to defuse tense confrontations
- improving the practice organisation so that the service provided is efficient
- devising a practice policy to handle a violent or aggressive incident
- equipping staff with assertiveness and anger management skills
- offering support to staff who have been victims of attack or abuse
- learning from any violent episode and making changes to avoid a recurrence.

The problem of aggression and violence suffered by those working in the
NHS is common in many workplaces, with around 35 000 staff being
attacked at their workplaces in the UK each year. Staff in medical
establishments are particularly vulnerable to aggression and violence:
they have a great deal of daily one-to-one contact with patients who are
mentally ill or disturbed, in circumstances where emotions run high and
normally sane patients or relatives can suddenly become irrational or
aggressive. Practice and community nurses, GPs and other healthcare staff
who visit patients in their own homes are often unaware of danger, because
their caring nature and their role as the patients' advocate makes them
unsuspicious of danger.

Even if they have never experienced actual violence themselves, most GPs
know of vicious attacks on other doctors and nurses and have been the
victim of verbal abuse and physical threats at some time in their career. All
this creates an atmosphere of fear for their personal safety on home visits,
especially amongst female GPs and practice staff.

Although the usual duty of doctors and healthcare staff is to provide care and uphold patient confidentiality, abuse and violence from a patient cancels this contract. Guidance from the General Practitioners Committee (formerly the General Medical Services Committee) firmly advises any victim to break confidentiality as regards name and contact details and make an official complaint to the police about any violent or threatening incident.[1]

Under-reporting of violent episodes is said to be widespread and people have different perceptions about behaviour which they class as threatening or offensive. Sometimes practice staff may tolerate particular patients' rudeness or threats and accept them uncomplainingly as a way of life. So GPs may only find that they have a problem with patients' rudeness and aggression in the practice if they ask staff directly about it.

Verbal abuse is thought to be at one end of a continuing spectrum that ends in physical assault. Such episodes should be treated seriously and not dismissed as trivial just because they were not accompanied by physical attack.

←—————————————————————————————————→

Verbal abuse   Threats/gestures   Physical contact (pushing, etc.)   Attack

The victim(s) of any violent incidents in the practice or on home visits should be encouraged to talk about their experiences and be debriefed as soon as possible after the event, or stress will invariably result. There should be a practice policy in place that everyone is familiar with, to reduce the likelihood of aggression and violence flaring in the practice, to defuse any such incident effectively, to summon help as necessary, and to counsel and support any victim afterwards.

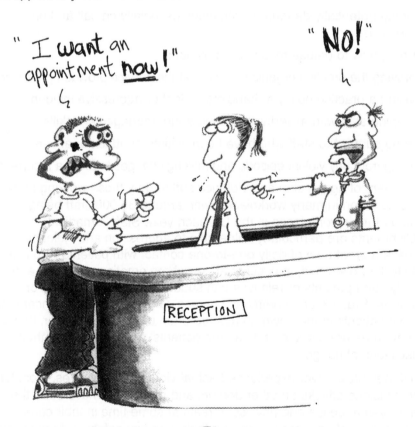

Avoiding aggression.

Avoiding circumstances that lead to aggression and violence

Violent behaviour can flare up in any practice unexpectedly, even in those with surgeries in pleasant, middle-class areas. But being able to recognise early warning signs of aggression and being more aware of risky situations should allow GPs and their staff to be better prepared to disarm anger and defuse potentially violent situations.

The practice should have a policy for dealing with verbal abuse and violence to which all doctors and staff should adhere. Sometimes a particular patient may behave well with some of the staff but be aggressive or abusive to others; whatever action is taken against the patient should have the full backing of all the GP partners, even those who have not been abused or witnessed bad behaviour. There is a distinction to be made between those patients who behave badly of their own volition and those who are temporarily mentally disturbed, as for example with a psychosis. Medical staff who are assaulted by a psychotic patient as part of their illness may rightly be more tolerant and not remove the patient from their list or prosecute him or her, but treat the patient instead.

Physical violence against GPs occurs more frequently during out-of-hours calls than at any other time, although a significant number of GPs, especially women doctors, fear personal attack on home visits carried out during the daytime too. The mushrooming of GP co-operatives with drivers accompanying the visiting doctors has solved much of the stress of on-call work for an increasing number of GPs – by reducing the frequency of on-call duty as well as providing more personal protection. But still many GPs are doing their own on-call armed only with a mobile phone accepting calls directly from patients; this has the great disadvantage that no-one else may know the location of the GP's visits and if he or she gets into difficulties and is assaulted inside a home, no-one will have any idea of their whereabouts. So every GP and nurse should work to a system whereby someone else has a record of the details of the timing and addresses of their home visits.

GPs as employers have an obligation to protect their staff in accordance with the Health and Safety at Work Act (1974). In the primary care context this means that the GPs, or the practice manager as their deputy, are required to identify the risks of violence or attack on staff and minimise those risks by providing appropriate training and safety measures. The Suzy Lamplugh Trust trains primary care staff in personal safety, organises workshops and sells a training resource pack and reference material to help employers run training sessions themselves.[2]

Self-defence courses may teach new skills which would only be used as a last resort. It is worth carrying out a regular review of potential risks to staff and their personal security. Episodes of aggression or violence occurring in the practice should be monitored and whoever in the practice is responsible for the policy or reports of incidents should see if any new measures could be introduced to avoid a similar situation recurring. Use an incident report sheet for every episode of violence or aggression and record the circumstances of the event, the probable reasons and any changes that were made to reduce the chances of a repeat performance. Review all incident record forms at least annually to look for trends and patterns and reconsider your security arrangements for staff and premises.

Patients can be expected to become aggressive and frustrated if the practice is disorganised, as for example when they have long waits to be seen, urgent appointments are not available, their notes or test results are lost and staff are offhand or disinclined to give patients the explanations they want. Waiting longer than expected is a potent catalyst for patient aggression. Thus improving the organisation of the practice so that it runs smoothly and efficiently should reduce the likelihood of aggression or violence flaring at the front desk or in the surgery.

One of the reasons patients become aggressive is if they feel that no-one is listening and they are unable to get their point across. The design of the reception desk should provide a balance between some security and protection for the receptionists without the appearance of a barrier to the patients. It is helpful to have a quieter spot to one side of the reception desk for interviewing a disruptive or aggressive patient out of view of the full waiting room of patients but still within earshot and help of other practice staff. A well-advertised practice complaints system should offer an official channel through which patients can vent their frustration if they are dissatisfied with some aspect of the practice care, as an alternative to their dissatisfaction boiling over into verbal or physical abuse of the staff.

Other receptionists nearby should be watching out for their colleagues to offer support at the first signs of trouble. This could mean, for instance, the staff alerting GPs to patients entering the surgery in a drunk or aggressive state. Rather than risk their being alone with a GP or practice nurse in a consultation room, it may be best to see them quickly in a corner of the waiting room and send them off the premises as soon as possible to be seen properly another day when they are behaving better. Staff can code the medical records envelope of certain patients with whom the women GPs or practice nurses feel uncomfortable or under threat, to indicate they should only be seen by one of the male partners or with a chaperone, so that these patients don't turn up for a consultation unexpectedly and take the doctors or nurses by surprise.

It is worth paying attention to the comfort of the surgery premises. Waiting to be seen may be made less arduous for patients if the lighting is good, soft music is calming, toys distract the children, or a public phone allows patients to notify others at home or work if they have been delayed, etc.

Unfortunately, even in reasonably happy practices aggression sometimes erupts between staff. Such incidents usually arise when communication in the team is poor and the management is weak. Interpersonal conflicts can create a lot of passion and the cause of the dispute needs to be sorted out quickly and resolved before the rest of the practice team divide into two factions supporting either party.

Sometimes receptionists try too hard to please the patients by fitting them in to be seen and creating extra appointments that overload the doctors. This scenario can create a flashpoint where the GP protests about the extra patients added on unexpectedly, storms into the reception area and vents his or her rage in full view of the waiting patients. To avoid this situation, ways to manage extra patients need to be agreed in advance at a practice meeting and everyone must abide by the agreed policy. Receptionists need to learn to be more assertive with patients so that they are not bullied into adding patients on as 'emergencies' for trivial complaints.

GPs and their staff are only human and are also going to be more stressed and irritable at times. Practice staff should be aware that GPs are going to be far more irritable and tired after a night on-call, or during the days they are covering emergencies or are particularly worried about problem patients. If staff can make allowances for when GPs are under par and try to shield them at these times from extra work or interruptions that could easily wait, tempers are less likely to be frayed. Similarly GPs need to be aware that it is a hard and often thankless job out there on the reception desk and to resist the temptation to make extra demands on the staff or to overreact when a small mistake is made, especially at peak surgery times.

GPs often misdirect their anger and frustration on to the wrong people. The receptionist may be in the firing line when they add to the GP's load by handing him or her another seemingly inappropriate request for a house call. The GP directs his or her anger to the message-taker rather than at the real cause of the problem.

Disarming anger is a necessary intervention at any stage from tension onwards. It is particularly useful early on when someone is telling you off, or a patient has started a tirade about a particular member of staff or some aspect of the practice organisation. First, the patient's anger should be simply acknowledged ('I can see you are very angry'), followed by an invitation to say what is troubling them and showing that they will be listened to. Even if the staff are frightened or becoming tense themselves they should adopt a normal voice and relaxed body language to create a calming effect on the angry person to defuse the confrontation. Repeating back to the patient what has just been said ('active' listening) demonstrates to the patient that what they've said and are feeling has been heard and noted ('I can see how angry ... must have made you feel'). Staff should apologise if they or the practice organisation is in error. To be most effective staff should then move on to try and resolve the conflict or find out more about the problem, if that is appropriate, calling on the practice manager to help if appropriate. Give the angry patient some idea of your intentions and how and when they will hear a report back.

How you say things is more important than what you say. Staff need to appear confident and assertive but not aggressive and they should be aware of the messages given out by their body language from the very first moment of the patient acting in an aggressive way. Normally, staff would put patients at their ease anyway. Defusing tension by remaining calm and unhurried is really just an extension of their normal manner.

The value of early counselling after a violent incident has been proven by reducing the amount of sick leave a 'victim' takes. There should be someone in the practice who will take responsibility for listening to and supporting the person who has been attacked or upset by another's aggression – probably the practice manager or one of the GPs. Their post-traumatic stress will be lessened by good support from others in the practice and by the knowledge that the GPs will try to reorganise the practice in some way to reduce the chance of a recurrence.

Tips for avoiding violence and aggression from patients whilst doing home visits

- Don't enter a house without an escort, preferably the police, if you suspect the possibility of violence.

- Stay nearest the door – leave it open for a speedy escape.

- If you feel insecure, switch your mobile phone on before you enter the house and arrange for someone at the practice or at home to listen in whilst you are inside. They can summon help quickly.

- Withdraw quickly at any signs of danger. Don't be brave or foolhardy. If there's a knife about leave if you can.

- Carry your medical equipment in your pockets or an inconspicuous bag.

- Ask the caller to ensure good lighting from their house, with the upstairs curtains drawn open, to enable you to find it more easily if it is dark.

- Don't curtail the telephone request until you have gained crystal clear instructions of how to find the house. Mark house numbers on your local maps, especially if the numbering is illogical.

- Be polite, courteous and non-aggressive however frustrated and angry you feel inside.

Preventing violence in general practice: a summary of official guidance for GPs[1]

1 Ensure your own behaviour is beyond reproach and does not contribute to the development of an abusive or violent incident.

2 Agree a written practice policy on the procedures to be followed when dealing with unreasonable patients that all GP partners adhere to.

3 Include your practice policy for dealing with threats or incidents of violence in your practice leaflet.

4 Be careful of your appearance when making house calls so that you are not conspicuous.

5 Develop good relations with your local police and invite them to accompany you on all visits or consultations where there appears to be a threat of violence.

6 Urge your local authority to improve street lighting and numbering.

7 Consult a reputable firm for advice on improving the security of your premises.

8 Do not be afraid to demonstrate your determination to initiate a criminal prosecution.

9 Carry a personal alarm in your hand or on your wrist – either a recently tested gas or battery noise alarm or one of the new extremely offensive odour anti-attack repellants (RAPEL).

Handling the aftermath of aggression and violence: summary of official guidance[1]

1 Always report the violent or threatening incident to the police and make an official complaint.

2 Divulge the name and contact details of the abuser/assailant but maintain confidentiality of the medical aspects of the consultation.

3 Threats, words, abuse or behaviour that leave the victim in distress or in fear of violence constitute an 'offence' in a surgery. But this classification does not apply in a patient's home and GPs do not have the same protection against such behaviour there.

4 Consider a private prosecution in a magistrate's court if the police decline to prosecute the offender.

5 Removal of a violent or abusive patient from your practice list has immediate effect. Notify the Health Authority or Health Board by phone or fax, and follow up the request in writing. Inform the secretary of the LMC who can warn other doctors in the neighbourhood.

6 The Health Authority/Health Board should alert the patient's new GP about the event which has warranted the removal or reallocation and any past history of violence.

7 After a violent incident you can take out an injunction restraining the person from approaching your surgery premises or home or being present in any place to which you or a deputy might be called.

EXERCISE 8   Review the safety and security arrangements to prevent the likelihood of violence and aggression in your practice or to the individuals who work there, and for handling it most effectively if it does occur.

How does your practice measure up? Circle the types of systems or procedures that exist in your practice:

Before	After
Staff training	Support
Team approach	Report
Adequate staffing	Analyse
Secure premises	Discuss
Surgery alarms	Change systems
Good environment	Review policy
Good communication	Prosecute
Practice policy	
Planned interventions for different eventualities	
General awareness of danger	
Good practice organisation	
Culture of concern for staff	

What are the most dangerous situations for *you* at work and what changes can you make to minimise the chances of aggression and violence arising?

Potentially threatening situations	Intended changes
•	
•	
•	
•	

Encouraging assertiveness skills

References

1 General Medical Services Committee (1995) *Combating violence in general practice*. British Medical Association, London.

2 Bibby P (1995) *Personal safety for health care workers*. Commissioned by the Suzy Lamplugh Trust. Arena, Aldershot.

Other Reading

Clarke D (1989) *Stress management: assertion training*. National Extension College, Cambridge.

Cozens J (1991) *OK 2 talk feelings*. BBC Books, London.

Davies P (1996) *Personal power: how to become more assertive and successful at work*. Piatkus, London.

Denny R (1997) *Succeed for yourself: unlock your potential for success and happiness*. Kogan Page, London.

Jeffers S (1987) *Feel the fear and do it anyway*. Rider, London.

Palladino C (1994) *Developing self-esteem*. Crisp Publications, California.

Audio cassettes

Wendy Lloyd Audio Productions Ltd. For the twin tapes of 'Feeling good': 30 Guffitts Rake, Meols, Wirral L47 7AD. Tel: 0151 632 0662.

MODULE 4
Defining time management

AIMS

The aims of Module 4 are:

1 To increase GPs' repertoire of ways to practise time management.

2 To help GPs review their priorities and reallocate the proportions of their time spent on different activities accordingly.

3 To engage GPs in making action plans to improve their time management.

CONTENTS

The total time to work through the module depends on the amount of time the reader spends reflecting on how the information in the module applies to him or her, before completing the exercises. The total time for which postgraduate education accreditation might be sought is twelve hours (including time for reading and thinking and undertaking the daily activities logs and the significant event analyses).*

---

* GP participants could apply to their region's Director of Postgraduate General Practice Education for permission to submit one or more completed modules for postgraduate education accreditation. Approval of such an application will be at the Director's discretion and may require the support of a local GP tutor in arranging assessment. No assessment will be undertaken by the author or Radcliffe Medical Press.

Here's what some GP participants said they had gained from undertaking the first *Survival Skills for GPs* programme:

'It enabled me to use time on call effectively.'

'It forced me to make time to think around the subjects involved.'

'I had to find time to complete this programme but it was worthwhile and very educational.'

'It made me take time to appraise my situation and endeavour to improve the quality of my life.'

'It has made me make changes.'

'It has helped me organise myself better.'

'Lack of a time limit means that the programme can be lived with over a period of time.'

'It has helped to increase my insight and made me change the booked consultation times, when I've been thinking about it for years.'

KEY PRINCIPLES OF TIME MANAGEMENT

This workbook is all about being smarter about getting through your work. A certain degree of time pressure may be necessary for you to maintain interest and momentum in getting a job done. But too much pressure will tip you over the stress performance curve as discussed in Module 1, so that you and your work suffers.

One of the most common sources of stress cited by GPs is time pressure. The key to good time management is to:

- balance your work and leisure time

- prioritise how you spend your time – do not allow yourself or others to waste it

- control interruptions

- include time for thinking, doing, meeting and learning in your working day

- allow sufficient time for the unexpected

- delegate whatever and however you can

- not procrastinate but get on with essential tasks

- be assertive – learn to say 'No' often enough, to unnecessary work or taking on other peoples' jobs and tasks

- make effective decisions, and don't look back

- review significant problems and learn to manage time better to avoid those problems in future by making realistic action plans.

Balance your work and leisure time successfully

One of the secrets of a happy life is to get the balance of stress right. Some stress is healthy, too much is not! The object is to achieve just enough stress to encourage optimum performance and enjoyment, but not so much as to make work seem an endless grind and impair performance.

One of the ways to reduce stress is to timetable enough free time during your day to have time for rest and relaxation to counteract the stresses and strains of your working life.

Try and complete work activities within the normal working day so that you have enough time for non-work-related activities in your life. If you do not allow sufficient time for leisure you will not have the opportunity for personal growth outside primary care and will probably become stale. You might set a target periodically to learn or improve at something outside work or take definite measures to nurture your relationship with your spouse, family and friends.

The best options are solutions that make time and space for you for fun, relaxation, hobbies and enjoying simple pleasures throughout your life as a stress-proofing measure, rather than suddenly adopting these methods to beat stress at one particular time in your working life. One of the best ways to monitor whether you are managing to keep enough protected time for yourself is to keep a daily activities log for a week or so. At a recent meeting the lecturer asked her medical audience to be honest and indicate how many of them had spent any time at all in the previous week pursuing an activity that was for their own enjoyment. Only a quarter of the audience could say that they had, which was a sad state of affairs (although it may be that the sort of doctors who go to such meetings are not representative of doctors as a whole!).

EXERCISE 1   Keep a log of daily activities for a week.

Photocopy the daily log and record all your activities each day for a week, including an off-duty period if possible. Sort the activities into three separate columns:

- *personal needs*, including shopping, sleeping, domestic chores, bodily needs, etc.

- *work,* including reading work-related books, journals and papers

- *leisure,* including sport, relaxation, reading, music, etc.

Work out totals of the types of activities for each day. Compare your daily recordings with the Health Education Authority's recommendations for a healthy lifestyle by grouping your activities in the same categories:

- 45–55% on personal needs

- 25–30% on work

- 20–25% on leisure.

When the work component increases above 25%, it is the leisure proportion of the day that is usually reduced.

Review of several days activities log

How do your totals compare with the Health Education Authority's guidelines? Enter your totals here:

- Personal needs:

- Work:

- Leisure:

Can you note any trends or patterns of activities – staying late at work, catching up on paperwork at home from your daily time logs?

Continued

EXERCISE 1   Continued.

Were you generally in control of the time spent on different activities in your days, or did events control you? *Yes, I was in control/No, events controlled me.*

What proportion of your days' timetables were your activities fixed (for instance, surgery or clinic times)? Write in how many hours are generally under your control each day where activities might be rescheduled in another way?

• Number of hours at work under your control:

• Number of hours outside work under your control:

What were the biggest time wasters for you?

• At work:

• Outside of work:

How much of your leisure time was spent doing what you wanted to do?

Were there any surprises arising from the daily time logs?

Do you need to make changes in your life to create more protected time for yourself (and family)? What do you intend to do and when?

Intend to	Start date
1	
2	
3	
4	
5	

Daily log of activities

TIME SPENT ON ACTIVITY (To nearest quarter of an hour):					
Personal needs (shopping, washing, domestic chores, sleeping)		**Work**		**Leisure**	
Activity	Time spent	Activity	Time spent	Activity	Time spent
	Total for day:		Total for day:		Total for day:

Prioritise your time: do not allow yourself or others to waste it

The first step is to be clear about your goals in your work and home lives, and leisure. How you allot your time will look very different if your main goal is to be a great golfer, or learn a new skill such as acupuncture, or to spend as much time as possible with your family. Plan your goals in association with whoever else they affect, and make sure that they don't conflict with each other if you have more than one goal.

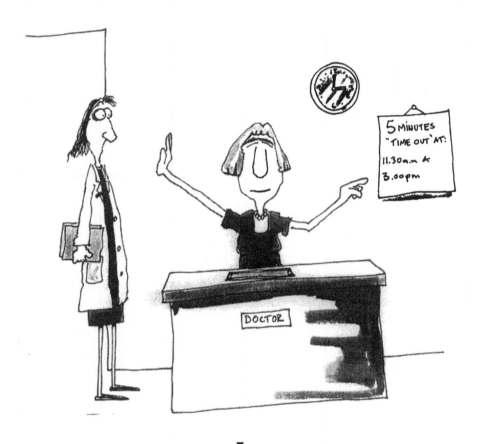

▼
Prioritise your time.

EXERCISE 2   Plan to achieve your goals.

1 *What goals do you want to achieve in the context of work?*

During this next month?

During this coming year?

2 *What goals do you want to achieve outside work?*

During this next month?

Over this coming year?

Set out your strategies for how you will achieve your goals.
What's hindering you? What will help you?

3 *What steps could you take to achieve your work goals*
(training, resources, set aside time, tasks, etc.)?

In the next month?

In the next year?

4 *What steps could you take to achieve your goals outside work*
(training, resources, set aside time, tasks, etc.)?

In the next month?

In the next year?

Now that you have your goals clear and have set out your strategies to achieve those goals you need to structure sufficient time around those priorities. Look back at the results of your week logging time spent on daily activities and map out the activities and tasks that are essential at work and home. Programme your priority activities in, either as a paper exercise or by thinking it through and resolving a new schedule.

When an activity arises and you have a choice about taking it on or not, match it against your goals. If it takes you further away from your goals, then refuse to take it on, but if it brings you closer to achieving your goals, consider if you have time to fit it in. Be firm with yourself and do not agree to do it just because you like the person who is asking you and want to please them – guard against being distracted by the hurly burly of general practice and distracted from your overall objectives.

Make sure that you spend your time doing the most important or complex jobs. It is too easy to focus on small, unimportant tasks and put off tackling the big ones, which just hang over you and make you feel guilty for being left unattended.

A high-priority task has to be done, a medium-priority job may be delegated and a low priority task should only be done if you have no medium- or high-priority tasks waiting, or you are too jaded to tackle them.

EXERCISE 3   Work out a timetabled programme to achieve the goals that you have just set for achieving at work and outside work.

Goal 1 Your work goal you want to achieve by the end of a month
What, when, how, where?

How will you know you have achieved your goal?

Goal 2 Your work goal you want to achieve by the end of the year
What, when, how, where?

How will you know you have achieved your goal?

Goal 3 Your goal for outside work that you want to achieve by the end of a month
What, when, how, where?

How will you know you have achieved your goal?

Continued

Control interruptions

Interruptions are one of the biggest time wasters, especially if someone else could have handled the problem or taken the message, or no action was required. Even if an interruption is necessary it may occur at the wrong time, wrecking your concentration or train of thought. Work out a system (and keep to it!) for letting others know when you are not to be disturbed and are spending time on priority tasks, and when you have an 'open door' and are available to deal with the queries that have built up whilst you were occupied. Keep focused on your priorities and don't allow others to engage you in chat when you intend to work. Agree rules in the practice for who may be interrupted and when. GPs become very stressed by incessant telephone interruptions whilst seeing patients; practice nurses bristle if staff constantly invade the treatment room to fetch equipment whilst they are treating patients; reception staff may lose track of their paper or prescription tasks if they keep breaking off to answer phone calls or find notes.

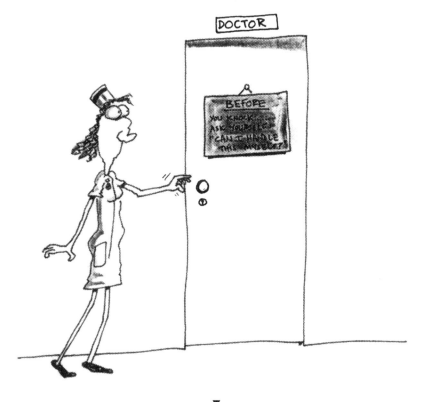

▼
Control interruptions.

EXERCISE 4   Tackle interruptions.

Which interruptions plague you most? Are they necessary?
You should be able to think of ways to minimise them effectively.

• Write down what is the most *frequent* interruption you receive at work.

• How could you minimise this kind of interruption occurring and/or its effect on you?

• So what changes will you make now?

• Write down what is the most *annoying* interruption at work.

• How can you minimise this kind of interruption occurring and/or its effect on you?

• So what changes will you make now?

Include sufficient time for thinking, doing, meeting, developing and learning

You need to be fresh and creative to stay on top of the demands in primary care and remain productive. You can only manage this in the longer term if you have the right mix of stimulating work, personal and professional development, and networking timetabled regularly into your daily schedule. Persistent overwork will be counterproductive and lead to negative stress and being less effective.

You will achieve more in designated sessions of quiet, uninterrupted time than in several times longer of fragmented time. This is the time for planning, writing reports or analysing progress.

Allow at least 10% of your time for dealing with unexpected tasks. In general practice it is reasonably predictable that you will have unexpected work to do. In the unlikely event that everything goes smoothly and you do not need the extra time, it will be a bonus to have that additional space to catch up on the backlog of paperwork.

You will have your own preference for thinking time, which to some extent will depend on your personality. Extroverts will be revitalised from brainstorming and discussions with a group of others, whilst those who are more introverted will prefer protected space in which to reflect and read. Whichever you prefer, make sure you get enough of it to replenish your creativity and enthusiasm. Some GPs join Balint groups with a few like-minded GPs to discuss practice problems. Learning sets are springing up offering development and support in small groups of peers of the same or different disciplines. Co-tutoring is an alternative to mentoring, and those who find a compatible co-tutee describe the benefits of having a buddy to listen to each other, and exchange ideas and support.

EXERCISE 5   Consider whether you are spending enough time on personal and professional development.

- When did you last clear enough space in your diary during working hours to *think* about anything developmental?

- Are you satisfied with the amount of time you have for personal and professional development?

- If you are dissatisfied, how can you clear space in your diary to attend an educational event on something you want to learn, meet with colleagues to discuss a special interest, find a co-tutee and set up a series of meetings?

- When will you start to timetable this in?

- What will you stop doing to accommodate this developmental time for yourself?

- What arrangements will you have to make to protect this self-development time?

Delegate whatever and however you can

Decide what only *you* can do and delegate as much as possible of the rest. It is important to remember this after the transition to primary care groups to reduce duplication between groups in a district for any tasks that can be core to all groups. Similarly, within a primary care group or within a practice, slim down the work as far as possible so that different disciplines are not doing the same work in parallel.

Delegate as much paper-based work as possible – it makes economic sense to ensure that there is sufficient clerical infrastructure to maximise clinical time. Use a dictaphone to record instructions about jobs that need doing or messages that need passing on, as well as letters for the secretary, and save time by delegating phone calls or dictating memos.

You should not just consider delegation at work, but at home too. General practitioners often find it difficult to relinquish control, and like to be seen as achieving in all spheres of their lives – super doctor/nurse, super homemaker, super parent, super spouse, etc. Well, it is perfectly alright to minimise the chores at home when you are so busy at work, and GPs often need 'permission' to do so. Employing domestic or gardening help is often cited by GPs as one of the most effective stress-relieving actions they have found, giving them instant access to time at home.

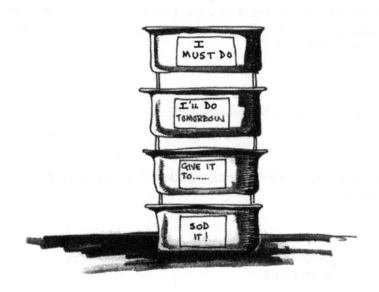

▼
Prioritise and delegate.

EXERCISE 6   Consider whether you are delegating work effectively and appropriately.

At work:

• Could you delegate work more than you do?

• Who could you delegate more to?

• What is stopping you delegating more work?

• What arrangements will you make to delegate more work?

• When and how?

At home:

• Could you delegate work more than you do?

• Who could you delegate more work to?

• What is stopping you delegating more work?

• What arrangements will you make to delegate more work?

• When and how?

Don't procrastinate: get on with essential tasks

So what are you waiting for? Distasteful or complicated tasks are the ones people procrastinate over. But if it is an essential or important task you will have to do it sometime, and you will only feel guilty putting it off. If you procrastinate too long the job will be even more difficult, as you will forget your previous ideas or what the instructions were. If you train yourself to do the least-wanted task first, you can reward yourself with a more pleasing job or even free time.

Wait until you have time to complete a stage or the whole of a job. Don't pick up a piece of paper and half read it, decide it is too difficult to tackle or you haven't enough time, and put it down again. You will have wasted that time deciding to put it off. And if you are in this procrastinating state of mind you may welcome unnecessary interruptions and compound the time wasting further. Try and get some momentum going and launch into it.

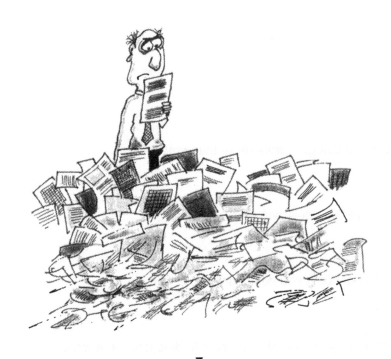

▼

Don't procrastinate.

Control your work flow

As well as using the control techniques described above, you should review the flow of your work to match your capacity. You are more likely to be most productive with a steady flow of work than a pressure/slack/pressure sandwich. If, in a practice, the surgery times mean that there is dead time in the middle of the day when you are less productive because the pressure is off and you waste time by taking longer to do little tasks, then find you work late in a pressured way, you will have to find ways as a practice to change the work flow in the system to suit you better. This might be by changing booking times, moving evening meetings to earlier slots in the day, etc.

Concentrate on one task at a time. Complete it and either move on to another job or take a short break to refresh yourself and clear your mind ready to start again. Don't move from one task to another or you will waste effort, having to start thinking about the topic all over again each time you take it up.

If you are swamped by work you will be less efficient and more forgetful, which may create even more time pressure if you have to put right the problem caused by you not remembering something or missing an appointment. You are likely to be more efficient if you group small, similar tasks together, such as returning phone calls. Always have one or two small jobs put by, or carried with you, so that if you are kept waiting you can get on with those jobs and not waste time.

Maintain control of your paperwork. Don't let it build up so that you feel overwhelmed or you will put off tackling it at all, or work more slowly as the enormity of the task depresses you. Insurance reports for completion by GPs are a good example. They have to be done. Some of the information can be completed by employed staff, but the more complex or interpretative sections require a clinical opinion. Why have them hanging over you for

---

days or weeks on end – you may as well set yourself a two- or three-day deadline to clear them, and they will seem less of a chore if they are not part of a mountain of paperwork.

Limit the time you spend on the telephone. If you time yourself the next few times you are on the phone you will probably be surprised how many minutes the calls last for. Listen to yourself and you may find that much of the time is spent on pleasantries or repeating yourself.

EXERCISE 8   Are you in control of your work, or does it control you?

- Do you control your work as much as possible, or do you let the work control you?

- What changes could you make to control the flow of your work in line with the ideas described above?

- When will you start?

- What will you do?

- Will these changes have any knock-on effects on you or anyone else?

Be assertive: say 'No' to unnecessary work or other peoples' jobs and tasks

The biggest challenge is to be assertive with yourself so that you don't agree to take on additional tasks that are not essential for you to undertake or that fall outside your own priority areas. If you are not careful you may be so busy helping others you do not get your own work done.

Module 3 on dealing with assertiveness techniques will give you more detailed help. The chief points to remember about being assertive are:

1 Say 'No' clearly and then move away or change the subject. Keep repeating 'No' – don't be diverted.

2 Be honest and direct with everyone.

3 Don't apologise or justify yourself more than is reasonable.

---

4 Offer a workable compromise and negotiate an agreement that suits you and the other party.

5 Pause before answering a 'Yes' you'll regret. Delay your response and give yourself more time to think by asking for more information.

6 Be aware of your body language and keep it as assertive as possible. Match your tone to your words (don't smile if you are giving a serious message).

7 Use the 'broken record' technique, persistently repeat your message in a calm manner to someone who is trying to pressurise you to do something you don't want to do. Don't be side-tracked.

8 Show you are listening to the other person's point of view and giving them a fair hearing.

9 Practise expressing your opinion and rights rather than expecting other people to guess what you want.

10 Don't be too hard on yourself if you make a mistake – everyone is human.

11 Be confident enough to change your mind if that is appropriate.

12 It can be assertive to say nothing.

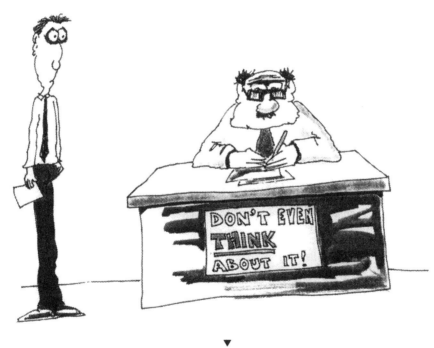

▼

Say 'No'.

Make effective decisions

Be decisive and finish jobs in hand. Gather information about a problem or choice, weigh up the pros and cons, and make a decision. Once you have made that decision look forwards and make plans for the future, don't look backwards and frame regrets. Some tips on making effective decisions are:

• There are always other options – find out what they are.

• Gather ideas and evidence from other people or a range of sources – do not be confined only to the options you already know about.

- Base your analyses and decision on reliable, objective evidence or observations, and not 'guesstimates'.

- Think through the implications of your decision by considering the possible consequences before choosing which options to take.

- Information is about feelings as well as facts – how the situation really is and how people feel about it.

- Your personality and beliefs will affect your decision-making process.

- Don't accept other people's perceptions of reality – look and think for yourself.

- Be honest with yourself and others, and keep your integrity – the best decisions are based on truth and not illusions.

- Effective decisions are based on reality and not hope.

- Probing questions help to distinguish between illusion and reality.

- Simple decisions are usually best, and often obvious, in retrospect.

- Fear gets in the way of making realistic assessments of the options.

- Don't make decisions because you are frightened of something, but because you are enthusiastic about the expected outcomes.

The more aware you are of your own character, the better you will understand how you make decisions. How you feel about how you make a decision often forecasts the results. If you feel good about a decision, the outcome is usually a success.

EXERCISE 9   Look at how good you are at making effective decisions.

- How good do you think you are in general about making effective decisions?

- What is stopping you being more decisive?

- How often do you regret a decision you have made? *Often/seldom/never*

- How often do you ruminate over decisions, going over and over again whether you did the right thing? *Often/seldom/never*

Continued

EXERCISE 9 Continued.

Describe an important decision you have to make now or in the near future:

• What are the options?

• What are the circumstances or potential advantages of your preferred option?

• What are the circumstances or potential disadvantages of your preferred option?

• What other information do you need to find out before making your decision?

• How sure are you that you have all the information possible, and have thought through the consequences of your decision for yourself and other people?

• If you have decided not to make any decision in the short-term, when will you review the situation?

• How much do you expect your decision to be a positive choice rather than one that makes the best of things?

• Is there any other way you could be more effective about making this decision?

EXERCISE 10   Which time management techniques have worked for you in the past?

Which do you still do? Tick which principles work for you in the table below.

Time management principles	Tried in past	Use now	Work for you
Keep time log of activities and review			
Write down tasks – prioritise and make an action plan			
Reduce unnecessary activities			
Get work in perspective and limit time spent			
Delegate appropriately			
Go on a formal course – time for reflection			
Whenever possible handle one piece of paper once – deal with it straight away			
Say 'No' to extra work			
Don't take on other peoples' jobs/tasks			
Set aside 'thinking' time			
Allow time for unexpected tasks (10%?)			
Be brief on the phone			
Tackle one task at a time – finish it			
Prepare for meetings to be effective			
Listen carefully to act correctly first time			
Don't procrastinate – do it now			
Do difficult tasks when most alert			

MAKE ACTION PLANS TO MANAGE YOUR TIME BETTER

Undertaking a significant event analysis of a frequently occurring time management problem or an unexpected crisis is a good way to work out the basis for a timetabled action programme to manage time better for you as an individual, or your practice team.

Read through the example below, and then work through two significant event analyses yourself – of you as an individual, and as one of a practice team if you cannot persuade the rest of your team to join in too.

Example of introducing an intervention to reduce the stress of telephone interruptions to GPs during surgery

Stage 1

Time stress topic chosen = reducing telephone interruptions in surgery.

This is an intervention concerned with preventing time stresses upon individual GPs.

Reason for choice = because telephone interruptions are a frequent cause of stress to GPs.

It seemed in this example as if such interruptions occur at least 10 times every surgery before the GPs set about recording whether this was really the case.

Stage 2

The standard might be: telephone interruptions during surgeries will only be made when patients phone for an emergency visit or another doctor phones and cannot be contacted easily after the surgery has finished. The standard should be set by all the GPs and agreed by the practice manager and practice staff.

Stage 3

Everyone agrees to the plan. No new skill training is needed. The new arrangements are to be a well-advertised, 30 minute time slot after surgery when patients and others can speak directly to a GP.

Their action plan is:

1 Agree standards with GP partners – no telephone interruptions other than from medical colleagues who are not easily contactable later on and from patients requesting emergency visits during surgery.

2 Seek agreement for proposed standards with receptionists and practice manager.

3 Nominate project leader (practice manager in this case).

4 Decide how the new system will operate (GPs and practice staff).

5 New system agreed to be 30 minute telephone contact time at the end of morning surgeries with all GPs.

6 Inform all GPs and practice staff of start date for new system of giving phone advice/speaking to GPs.

7 Put a notice up in the waiting room to inform patients that the trial system is running.

8 Expected outcome(s):

   (i) Advantage: GPs will feel less time pressured during surgery consultations.
   (ii) Disadvantage: GPs may be delayed after surgery waiting for 30 minute phone contact time to expire.

Stage 4

Prepare data recording forms, photocopy and distribute.

Stage 5

Collect baseline information. All GPs to record how many times they are interrupted during each surgery for one week before the new system is introduced. The recording should also note how many of the interruptions are from medical colleagues or patients requesting emergency visits during surgeries.

Stage 6

Start new system of telephone contact time. During the week after the new system is introduced, all GPs to record the number of and reason(s) for telephone interruptions during surgeries and throughout telephone contact times. (See example of data collection form on p. 105 for one GP recording number and reasons for telephone interruptions per weekday.)

Stage 7

Project leader compares GPs' results as aggregated anonymised comparison of the week's recordings of numbers and reasons for telephone contacts after the new system was introduced compared to:

(i) before the new system was introduced

(ii) the standards set at the beginning of the project.

Stage 8

Feed back these comparative results to all GPs and practice staff. (In this case, performance was better than before the new system was introduced when there were as many as 10 phone interruptions per surgery, but not as good as the agreed standards as there were still some phone calls that were not about emergency visits or from medical colleagues that were being put through to the GP, according to the data collection recording chart.)

Review of outcomes:

(i) Advantages of new system:

- GPs less time pressured and consequently feel less stressed without so many interruptions.

- GPs able to concentrate on seeing patients without being distracted by interruptions.

- GPs less likely to make mistakes during surgeries, e.g. prescribing errors, forgetting to refer patients, with fewer interruptions occurring.

(ii) Disadvantages of new system:

- Patients may be unaware of the new system and so phone in twice as much – first to try to speak to the GP during surgery time, and second to make the postponed call.

- GPs might leave the surgery a few minutes later to do house calls if delayed by the telephone contact time.

- Occasionally, GPs might have to wait for patients to come down to surgery after speaking on the phone whereas if the call had been taken earlier the patient might have been slotted in during surgery time.

Further changes might be:

(i) To advertise the new system of telephone contact time to patients by posters, word of mouth, practice leaflet. Otherwise the practice staff will end up being more stressed by the extra telephone calls and the patients' aggravation at being even less able to get though to the practice on the telephone.

(ii) To reinforce the importance and benefits of the new system to the GPs and practice staff, to further improve performance and try to reach the agreed standard.

Stage 9

Monitor one month later by GPs recording the number and type of interruptions for a few days, especially to ensure that patients are not abusing the easy telephone access to GPs by phoning to discuss trivial matters.

Example of daily data collection form

Number of interruptions and reasons one week after new system introduced

Weekday (Monday/ Tuesday /Wednesday/Thursday/Friday)

Morning surgery:	111
Afternoon surgery:	Not in surgery
Evening surgery:	11
Type of phonecall:	
• medical colleague	1
• emergency visit request	1
• not medical colleague and not emergency	120

EXERCISE 11   Undertake an analysis of a significant event involving a time management problem at work for you as an individual.

Focus on analysing the significant event from the perspective of preventing the time management problem for you as an *individual*. Your aim will be to reduce or change the nature of the time stressor; to remove the 'hazard' or reduce the frequency/extent of the time stressor. If prevention is impossible, a secondary approach would be to alter the ways in which you as an individual respond to the time stressors, or improve your ability to recognise and deal with time-related problems as they arise.

Stage 1

Write down a factual account of the time pressured situation you have chosen – who was involved, what time of day, what task/activity you were doing. The situation should be a frequent source of time stress, an important cause of time stress or an infrequent event that when it occurs has far-reaching effects, or a time stress which is costly in terms of time or resources; it must be a realistic choice, i.e. a cause of time stress which you can reasonably expect to be able to reduce.

Stage 2

Set a 'standard' or a sensible target to aim at that is a recognisable measurement of an acceptable reduction in the time stress you hope to achieve after you have introduced a new system to reduce the cause of that stress. You may need to carry out baseline data collection first to provide sufficient information to set the standard if there is no obvious reference point. Record the effects of this cause of time stress on you.

Stage 3

Write out a plan to reduce the time pressure, including the expected outcomes and the expected benefits and disadvantages. Discuss your proposal with everyone else involved, at home and at work. Obtain the agreement of anyone who may be concerned by the proposed changes to your set standard(s) and your proposed intervention(s). Amend your plans in the light of others' comments.

Stage 4

Prepare to carry out your plan. This will include obtaining or buying any extra equipment, training yourself or others if new skills are required, applying for extra staff time or making other resource or organisational arrangements.

Continued

EXERCISE 11 Continued.

Stage 5

Record current performance as a baseline before making any changes. The data collection form on p. 108 may be helpful at this stage. Fill in your own row and column headings as appropriate for your project.

Stage 6

Introduce and carry out the intervention, e.g. starting the new system or beginning to use new equipment. Record new performance measures.

Stage 7

Compare new performance with old performance, and with pre-set standards. Has the agreed standard been reached?

Stage 8

Feed back information about comparison of performance (i.e. Stage 6 results), outcomes of intervention(s) and the improvements or changes to those involved in, or affected by, the project. Discuss as a work team and agree and make further changes if standards were still not met. Arrange further training, etc. if current skills are still inadequate.

Stage 9

Monitor performance 3–6 months later. Reinforce interventions and/or changes as necessary.

Data collection form

Defining time management

EXERCISE 12   Undertake an analysis of a significant event involving a time management problem at work for you as a practice.

For this exercise, focus the analysis of the significant event from the point of view of preventing that time management problem in your *practice team* by reducing or changing the nature of the time pressure; removing the 'hazard' or reducing the frequency or extent of the time stressor. If prevention is impossible, a secondary approach would be to alter the ways in which you as a work team respond to the time stressors or improve your ability to recognise and deal with time-related problems as they arise.

Stage 1

Write down a factual account of the circumstances of the time pressured situation you have chosen to review – who is generally involved, the time of day and the task or activity concerned. The situation should be a frequent source of time stress, an important cause of time stress or an infrequent event that when it occurs has far reaching effects, or a time stress which is costly in terms of time or resources; it must be a realistic choice, i.e. a cause of time stress which you can reasonably expect to be able to reduce.

Stage 2

Set a 'standard' agreed with others from the practice or from published literature, or pick a sensible target to aim at that is a recognisable measurement of an acceptable reduction in the time pressure that you hope to achieve after you have introduced a new system to reduce the cause of that time stress. You may need to carry out baseline data collection first to provide sufficient information to set the standard if there is no obvious reference point. Write down the effects of time pressure on the participants in the crisis or stressful situation you have chosen.

Stage 3

Write out a plan to reduce the time pressure, including the expected outcomes and the expected benefits and disadvantages. Discuss and agree the proposal for change with everyone else involved at work. Obtain the agreement of anyone who may be concerned by the proposed changes to your set standard(s) and your proposed intervention(s). Amend your plans in the light of others' comments.

Continued

EXERCISE 12   Continued.

Stage 4

Prepare to carry out your plan. This will include obtaining or buying any extra equipment, training yourself or others if new skills are required, applying for extra staff time, or making other resource or organisational arrangements.

Stage 5

Record your team's current performance as a baseline before making any changes. The data collection form on p. 108 may be helpful at this stage. Fill in your own row and column headings as appropriate for your project.

Stage 6

Introduce and carry out the intervention, e.g. a new system or using new equipment. Measure your new performance.

Stage 7

Compare your team's new performance with their old performance and with pre-set standards. Has the agreed standard been reached?

Stage 8

Feed back information about comparison of your performance (i.e. Stage 6 results), the outcomes of the intervention(s) and the improvements or changes to those involved in, or affected by, the project. Discuss as a work team and agree and make further changes if the standards were still not met. Arrange further training, etc. if current skills still seem to be inadequate.

Stage 9

Monitor your team's performance 3–6 months later. Reinforce the interventions and/or changes as necessary.

EXERCISE 13   Complete a personal contract.

Specify three ways in which you intend to manage time more effectively in future:

What are the obstacles to overcome? What may stop you acting to manage time more effectively?

What will you do and when will you start?

Intended action	Start date
1	
2	
3	

Further reading

Clarke D (1989) *Stress management: time management section.* National Extension College, Cambridge.

Time management consultants

Hallam Management Services. Run workshops individualised for those working in primary care: 143 Green Oak Road, Sheffield S17 4FS. Tel: 0114 262 0959.

MODULE 5
Enhancing job satisfaction

AIMS

The aims of Module 5 are:

1 To increase awareness of the ingredients of job satisfaction amongst GPs.

2 To engage readers in making plans to actively promote job satisfaction.

3 To encourage a more positive outlook to working in general practice.

CONTENTS

Working in partnerships at work and outside work

    Exercise 18: Review features of your own partnerships (time = 20 mins)

    Exercise 19: To what extent are you satisfied with your job overall?
                 (time = 10 mins)

The total time to work through the module depends on the amount of time the reader spends reflecting on how the information in the module applies to him or her, before completing the exercises. The total time for which postgraduate education accreditation might be sought is six hours (including time for reading and thinking and completing all the exercises and plans).*

Here's what some GP participants at a professional development course said about their experiences:

'The course has developed my skills. It has allowed me to appreciate and enjoy aspects of general practice which had been overlooked before.'

'I have shifted towards finding time for my own interests instead of those of my family and this has given me increased satisfaction.'

'It was good to remember my reasons for doing general practice in the first place – good to be reminded of advantages.'

'I'll look to expand partner social activity rather than just work.'

'It's not classroom teaching but reflective.'

'The programme makes you think about your life.'

'The material has given me a greater understanding of my work/family life.'

---

* GP participants could apply to their region's Director of Postgraduate General Practice Education for permission to submit one or more completed modules for postgraduate education accreditation. Approval of such an application will be at the Director's discretion and may require the support of a local GP tutor in arranging assessment. No assessment will be undertaken by the author or Radcliffe Medical Press.

CHECKING OUT JOB SATISFACTION

Studies of the general public show that most workers rate job satisfaction and opportunities for learning, and personal and professional development more highly than job security or level of earnings. Job satisfaction helps to 'stress-proof' a person and protect them against stress resulting from excessive demands at work. If a person is satisfied and interested by their job, their motivation will help keep up standards of performance and the quality of their work.

One of the best ways to 'stress-proof' yourself against the stresses of a job is to explore and expand factors which give you the most job satisfaction. If you enjoy your job as a GP, feel in control of your everyday work and find many aspects of the job satisfying, this will minimise the effects of the parts of the job you find more stressful.

Women GPs seem to have greater job satisfaction than their male colleagues and the general population.

The four aspects of their work that give GPs most dissatisfaction are: demands of the job and patients' expectations, interference with family life, constant interruptions at home and work, and practice administration. For women GPs, it is the work/home interface that causes most dissatisfaction, and for men, the demands of the job and patients' inappropriate expectations.

The highest levels of satisfaction for male and female GPs are gained from the responsibility that comes with the job, being in control of how they work and the amount of variety in the job. Female GPs are more satisfied with their hours of work and rate of pay than their male counterparts and more likely to report that they enjoy their work. Another difference studies have noted between male and female GPs is that men find psychosocial aspects of general practice less satisfying, but managing and organising more rewarding, than women do.

Studies of GPs' job satisfaction have shown a downward trend since the late 1980s with regard to satisfaction from the amount of responsibility, variety in the job, physical conditions at work, amount of freedom to choose their own working methods and the recognition they receive for good work. The least satisfied GPs seem to be in the 35 to 44 year age group.

We know that lower rates of job satisfaction are associated with mental and physical ill health, levels of perceived stress and sick leave. Low job satisfaction can affect performance – one example is the link that has been shown between low job satisfaction and poor prescribing practice. Job satisfaction can be promoted through continuing professional education and development, and opportunities for career advancement.

EXERCISE 1   Reflect back on why you chose your particular career as a GP.

Think back and remember how and why you came to choose general practice rather than a career in other specialties. Did you make a positive choice or did you just drift into working in general practice because you thought it would be the most compatible with looking after and rearing a family? Or were there other complicating factors? Write down below all the positive reasons you had for making your career choice when you were younger. Mark against them if they still apply or whether circumstances have changed. Have you lost sight of the positive side of general practice that attracted you in the first place?

Reasons for choosing your job   Do they still apply?
in general practice

-

-

-

-

-

The spectrum of support and development for pursuing professional and job satisfaction

Continuing personal and professional development are integral with maintaining job satisfaction and professional fulfilment. The table below illustrates the possibilities of underpinning an individual's well being with education and support activities, and describes the broad picture of measures that can be adopted to enhance well being and fulfilment as a GP.

Serious health problems	Depression, anxiety	Well-being development	Professional fulfilment
Referral to specialist	Support systems	Stress management	Career development
Rehabilitation	Counselling	Team building	Well organised practice
		Communication	
		Assertiveness	Good job fit
		Time management	Rewards for performance
		Continuing education	Job appraisal
			Learning new skills, e.g. higher degree

EXERCISE 2   Do you spend sufficient time on education and support activities?

Hopefully you are either consciously or unconsciously competent at work as far as possible. The problem is that the focus on evidence-based practice has made people realise how little we do with regard to clinical work for which there is hard evidence, so that we may be unconsciously incompetent at work more often than we realise. Doctors who are burnt out or over-stressed may slip into conscious incompetence as they cut corners or ignore patients' emotional cues as a poor way of coping with patients' demands.

Are you satisfied with how you learn? Do you know what your preferred learning style is? Some people who prefer project work do best compiling a portfolio of new material, others prefer to read quietly by themselves, some prefer to attend lectures, not all of which are inspirational. If you are aware of your learning style you can choose educational events that suit you best.

Write down what activities you have actively sought or undertaken in the last month, that come under the umbrella of the type of activities described in the columns of 'well being' or 'career development' in the table on the previous page:

How much time have you spent on these education or support activities?

Do you think you have invested sufficient time in the last month developing your job and skills?

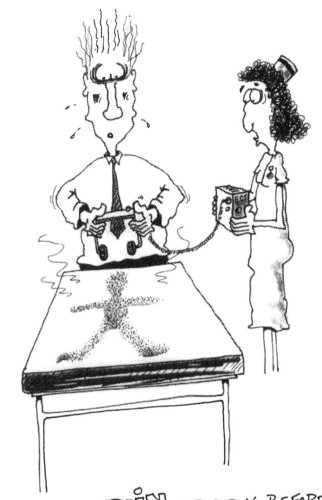

LEARN AND TRAIN PROPERLY BEFORE PRACTISING NEW SKILLS!

▼

Practice makes perfect.

EXERCISE 3   Find out what your sources of job satisfaction are and how they compare with other peoples'.

Complete the questionnaire below indicating what gives you most satisfaction at work. The factors are not in any order of priority and have been identified by other GPs as sources of satisfaction at work for them.

Please score each factor according to how important a source of satisfaction you think it is for you, from 'No satisfaction', to 'Moderately satisfying' or 'Very satisfying'. Please add alternative sources of satisfaction for you to the bottom of the table if they do not appear in the prepared list.

Source of satisfaction	How satisfying?		
	Not satisfying	Moderately satisfying	Very satisfying
Relationships with patients			
Ability to treat illness			
Relationship with practice staff other than GPs			
Relationship with other doctors (including partners)			
Financial security			
Own working conditions			
Public's view of the medical profession			
Ability to prevent illness by health promotion			
Other:			
Other:			

Now compare your answers with the results of a survey of 620 GPs from Staffordshire.[1] Responses from male and female respondents have been separated as there were some gender differences, so please look down the appropriate column to compare how your own results match up with how satisfying other GPs found each factor of their job. The majority of Staffordshire GPs found the top five factors in the table 'very satisfying'

Source of satisfaction	% of general practitioners					
	Male (n = 481)			Female (n = 139)		
	Not	Moderate	Very	Not	Moderate	Very
Relationship with patients	5	22	71	1	19	78
Ability to treat illness	5	23	70	3	19	76
Relationship with practice staff	7	31	60	5	25	68
Relationship with other doctors	10	29	54	11	24	63
Financial security	13	33	52	12	26	60
Own working conditions	20	31	47	16	42	40
Public's view of profession	44	34	18	42	42	15
Prevent illness by health promotion	62	22	13	57	27	16

Continued

EXERCISE 3   Continued.

How did you do?

Do you have other major sources of job satisfaction? If so, what?

1

2

3

EXERCISE 4   What sources of job satisfaction could you enhance (at least two)?

1

2

3

4

What action do you propose to take in relation to the sources of satisfaction you have just identified above, and when?

Action proposed	Start date
1	
2	
3	
4	

MOTIVATION

People are motivated by different things, and arguments rage as to whether anyone is ever driven by entirely altruistic motives. Some of the best motivators for fulfilling peoples' needs are:

- interesting and/or useful work

- sense of achievement

- responsibility

- opportunity for career progression or professional development

- gaining new skills and competencies

- sense of belonging to practice or primary care group.

A study of young people's work ethic has found that 'Generation X' (the 18 to 29 year age group) wants stimulating work, variety, to be constantly learning and receive continuous feedback on how they are doing.[2] Other studies of job satisfaction in organisations in general show that employees rate achievement, recognition, responsibility, advancement and growth more highly than salary, status, security, supervision, relationships with work colleagues and work conditions.

Pride, lust, anger, gluttony, envy, sloth and covetousness are all listed as prime motivators of people – hopefully not all of these are relevant to any great extent in the general practice environment. Money motivates many GPs and other self-employed health professionals, fuelled by the tradition of the NHS recompensing their work as item-of-service payments. The need for self-employed health professionals to make sure that their small businesses remain viable by focusing on assured income is much misunderstood by employed health professionals in other care settings.

If you are trying to set up a new scheme or project in a practice, you have to understand what motivates you and the others with whom you work if you want to build in motivating factors that will encourage their co-operation.

Maslow's hierarchy of a person's needs describes how self-esteem and fulfilment are not possible if the basic structure and safety components of your life are not secure.[3] Self-esteem encompassing self-respect, status and recognition from others are only possible if they are built upon a good social base that includes love, friendship, belonging to groups (work, home, leisure, professional) and social activities. Fulfilment, maturity and wisdom are only possible in a person where all the other conditions of their life encourage growth, personal development and accomplishment. Practice managers, GP employers and the NHS management in general have a responsibility to create a working environment in which motivation can take place and needs be met.

EXERCISE 5   What mainly motivates you?

Once you have achieved an income in your family unit that gives you a reasonable standard of living, what would you say you are mainly motivated by (e.g. money, helping people)? Write down the top three motivators that apply to you in relation to your job:

-

-

-

GET THE RIGHT BALANCE IN YOUR JOB

The following exercises consider features of work in general practice that doctors frequently identify as important aspects of their work and job satisfaction. Make an assessment of how satisfied you are with your current job by completing the exercises, reviewing the implications of your responses and making a plan if you can see there's a need to make changes.

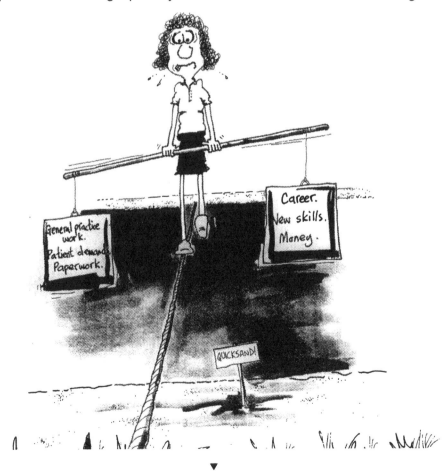

▼

Get the right balance in your job.

EXERCISE 6   Review how satisfied you are with the amount of money you earn (taking into account income earned by others with whom you live).

- Do you earn an appropriate amount for your or your family unit's needs?

Too much/Appropriate/Too little

Review: If you feel that you earn too much or too little, do you want to plan to increase or decrease your income?

So what's your plan?

- Are you content with the balance between the level of your income and free time? *Yes/No*

Review: Would you be prepared to reduce your income substantially for a corresponding gain in free time or slower work pace, or do you wish to increase your income with a corresponding reduction in your free time?

So what's your plan?

EXERCISE 7   Look at opportunities for professional development (at work).

- Do you have sufficient opportunities to learn new skills, undertake education, network with other like-minded colleagues? *Yes/No*

Review: If you do not have sufficient opportunities for professional development what do you need to do: create dedicated time, identify contacts or experts, find resources such as course fees, find sources of information describing a range of opportunities and how to progress?

So what's your plan?

- How motivated are you about pursuing professional development consistently? *Well motivated/Indifferent/Hostile to idea of continuing professional development*

Review: If you are indifferent or hostile to continuing professional development is it because you are stressed or burnt out, or do you feel that your performance cannot be bettered and there is nothing you don't know, or do you just never get round to prioritising time for professional development? Is there any way or any person with whom you can explore the underlying reasons for your not embracing a professional development culture? What about visiting a stress counsellor, GP tutor, time management specialist?

So what's your plan?

EXERCISE 8   To what extent do you use your skills, knowledge and experience?

• How often do you use the majority of your skills, knowledge and experience as a doctor or health professional? *Every day/Most days/ Once a week/Occasionally*

Review: In what ways might you use your skills, knowledge and experience better in your current workplace? Will it require substantial changes to make more use of your skills, knowledge and experience without moving outside your workplace? Will it be worth the effort of expanding your horizons and doing at least some work outside your workplace in order to make more use of your skills, knowledge and experience?

So what's your plan?

EXERCISE 9   How contented are you with the interpersonal relationships at work?

• Do you like your colleagues at work, do they like you? *Yes, usually/Indifferent/Actively dislike*

• To what extent do you need to feel liked by everybody? *Yes, usually/Indifferent*

Review: Does constantly aiming to be liked interfere with your feeling comfortable at work, and does it force you to behave unnaturally? If work colleagues dislike each other is there anything you can do to build a team spirit through group activities at work or social events outside work?

So what's your plan?

• To what extent do you respect your work colleagues and do they respect you? *Usually respect each other/One-sided respect/Mutually disrespectful*

Review: Are you content with the situation? Is there anything else you might do to build up your colleagues' respect for you, or at least to cease losing their respect?

So what's your plan?

EXERCISE 10   How reasonable is your workload?

- How does the level of demands making up your workload seem to you? *Too much/About right/Too little*

- Is there a good balance between the proportion that is boring or routine and stimulating or challenging? *Good balance/Poor balance*

- Is the workload distributed well throughout your working day? *Usually well distributed/Mixed or unpredictable*

Review: What else might be done to maintain your workload at reasonably consistent levels? How much of these alterations are within your control?

So what's your plan?

EXERCISE 11   How satisfied are you with your working hours?

- How satisfied are you with your working hours, the number of hours, timing? *Usually contented/Indifferent/Usually discontented*

Review: If you are discontented or think your working hours could be improved, what else might be done to achieve better working hours? How much of these changes is within your control?

So what's your plan?

EXERCISE 12   How satisfied are you with the degree of participation or control you have over your work?

- How satisfied are you with the extent to which you are involved in decision making at work? *Generally satisfied/Seldom satisfied/Not satisfied*

Review: If you are dissatisfied what else could you do to improve your involvement in decision making at any or all levels of the practice organisation?

So what's your plan?

- Does the practice have a mission statement, set of values or development plan? If so, do you know what they are?

Review: Are you as aware as you might be of what the intended direction of the practice is?

So what's your plan?

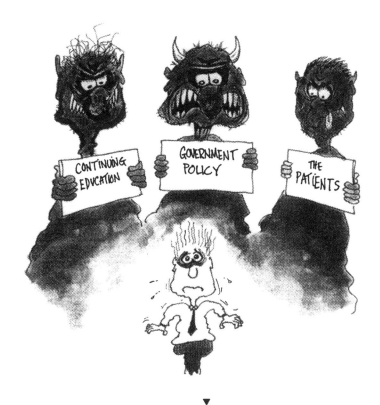

▼
Controlling your work.

EXERCISE 13   What opportunities do you have for additional work-related activities?

- Do you have the time to accommodate additional or interesting work outside the practice? *Easily have time/Difficult but possible to fit additional work in/Impossibly time-constrained*

- Are your work colleagues supportive about enabling you to fit other work into your practice timetable? *Supportive and facilitatory/Supportive but not actively facilitatory/Neither supportive nor facilitatory*

Review: If you have the inclination for additional work but do not have time, could you change the extent of your commitments at work by delegating a current task or responsibility, or ceasing to participate in an activity such as offering a special service or sitting on a committee? Could you convert reluctant partners to being supportive by profiling the advantages of any additional work you take on from your and their viewpoints? A happier and more fulfilled colleague should benefit them, even if there are no direct tangible advantages.

So what's your plan?

Continued

Enhancing job satisfaction   **127**

EXERCISE 13 Continued.

- Do you have the time to accommodate additional or interesting work as part of extended services offered by the practice? *Easily have time/Difficult but possible to fit additional work in/Impossibly time constrained*

- Are your work colleagues supportive about enabling you to fit new activities or services into your practice workload? *Supportive and facilitatory/Supportive but not actively facilitatory/Neither supportive nor facilitatory*

Review: If you have the inclination to extend the services offered by the practice but do not have the time, could you reorganise your practice commitments by delegating a current task or responsibility, or ceasing it altogether? Could you work out a way of convincing your colleagues that the benefits of the innovations and changes you propose outweigh potential disadvantages or risks?

So what's your plan?

- Do you have good information and awareness of the wide spectrum of jobs and activities that are available to practising clinicians? *Yes/No*

Review: If you are unsure or know that your information and awareness is limited, could you make more contacts in likely places, let others know you are available, search out adverts in journals or newspapers you don't usually read (such as management posts in associated journals or public service appointments advertised in national newspapers)?

So what's your plan?

EXERCISE 14   To what extent are you satisfied with the level of your core skills?

- What about new skills like your level of computer literacy? Do you have basic keyboard skills, i.e. type with more than two fingers? *Yes/Some/No*

- What are your communication skills like? Have you become increasingly paternalistic as you've become longer in the tooth? Can you switch into different consulting styles intentionally to suit the patient and the circumstances or are you stuck in a communication rut? *Good communicator/Fair communicator/ Poor communicator*

Review: There are many skills and competencies that once gained make your job easier and give you a sense of pride and achievement. Make a mental list now of what core skills you have and which you should try to learn. Here's an opportunity to resolve to learn those skills you have been meaning to get round to someday.

So what's your plan?

EXERCISE 15   How satisfied are you with your practice organisation?

- Does everything run smoothly? How satisfied are you with the way the practice is organised? *Very satisfied/Moderately satisfied/ Not at all satisfied*

- Is the practice well managed, with good employment practices, such as inductions for new staff, regular job appraisals for all staff, attention to healthy working and adequate staff training?

Review: For a well-ordered, meticulous person, there's nothing more frustrating than trying to work amidst chaos with notes misfiled, lost correspondence, meetings starting late, etc. Conversely, a disorganised person who lets medical records pile up in his or her car or a corner of the surgery, who forgets to pass on messages or turns up late for surgery, will wreck the arrangements in a well-managed practice and annoy the rest of the staff. Good management will depend on the GPs agreeing goals, policies and procedures for a smooth practice organisation delivering high-quality care and then trying to carry them out. And supporting the lead manager in applying and implementing those policies.

So what's your plan?

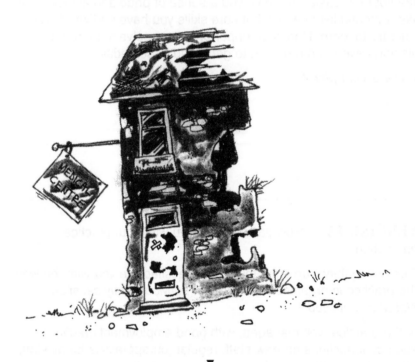

▼
Your environment.

EXERCISE 16   Check out your consulting room or usual work space and look at:

- Your chair – is it comfortable, is the backrest adjusted to your needs, can you alter the seat to the height that suits you and does it remain there without slipping down?

- Your desk – is it big enough, is it avoidably cluttered, is it in the best position?

- The lighting – is it adequate when it is dark outside, do you need extra lighting for carrying out examinations?

- The ventilation – do smelly feet, bad breath or unwashed bodies hang around? Can you improve the air flow or import a better background smell?

- The degree of privacy of your conversations – can you overhear the conversations in the surgery next door, or are you aware that your voice carries through to patients waiting outside your door? Would noise masking help?

- The noise outside – are your windows thick enough to exclude external noise sufficiently? Could you muffle it more by arranging different ventilation or adding secondary double glazing?

- Liquid refreshment – could you indulge yourself with drinks to hand, a small coffee machine, or a small fridge actually in your consulting room?

- The decor – does it need freshening up, a different colour scheme or new pictures?

- Trophies and treasures – do you have any on display to remind you of your past personal or professional achievements, favourite holidays, fond family memories, etc?

- Humorous touches – is there anything you can glance at when the going gets tough and you want to buck yourself up: pithy sayings, funny cartoons, witty books?

So, what's your plan? What changes will you make to your environment?

Note: there is no section or exercise on satisfaction with your current lifestyle and thinking about whether your quality of life is as good as you would wish because Module 4 focuses on time management and allocating sufficient time to the priorities in your life.

IMPROVING SATISFACTION WITH YOUR ENVIRONMENT

Working in a disturbing or unpleasant physical environment is likely to cause you stress and conversely, working in a restful, pleasing environment reduces stress.

EXERCISE 17   Identify some positive features of your working
and home lives.

Write down three examples from work which illustrate you having a
positive outlook on life (e.g. a recent achievement):

-

-

-

Write down three examples from outside work which illustrate you
having a positive outlook on life (e.g. pride in a skill such as sailing):

-

-

-

Is there anything you might do to think or behave in a more positive
manner more often (e.g. smile more):

-

-

-

DEVELOPING A POSITIVE ATTITUDE TO YOUR WORKING LIFE

Job satisfaction is very much to do with your attitude to work and your expectations. There may be many aspects of your work that you would eliminate or change if you had a free choice. Working with a group of other colleagues means making compromises so that you can work as a team, and the capacity to accommodate your personal preferences will depend on the size of the team and the power structure. When you cannot have things exactly the way you want them at work you can either be overly frustrated and chaff over the limitations, or you can develop the sort of attitude that makes the best of things with a generally positive outlook on life. Many GPs are suffering from 'change fatigue' after the succession of major reorganisations in primary care over the last decade; a positive outlook combats many of the frustrations resulting from so much change.

For a positive approach:

• concentrate on what you can do and not what you cannot do

• accept your limitations – you're not superwoman/superman/super housewife/husband/superspouse

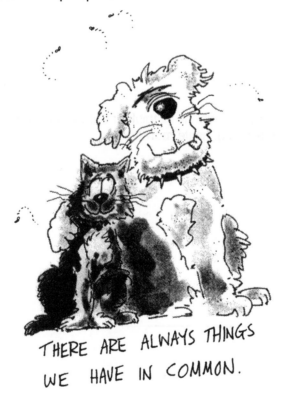

THERE ARE ALWAYS THINGS WE HAVE IN COMMON.

▼

Working in partnership.

• get things in perspective – don't get overwhelmed by demands; put problems and unhappy experiences behind you

---

BOX Features that encourage an effective partnership between individuals and/or organisations (adapted from Chambers and Lucking, 1998)[4]

- The partnership as a whole is greater than the sum of the components.

- A written memorandum of partnership exists, such as a contract, letter of agreement, etc.

- The partnership has a vision and plan for development.

- The partnership benefits both.

- There are mutually agreed goals and expected outcomes.

- The partnership has general wide support.

- There are clear roles and responsibilities with respect to joint working.

- There is shared decision making on partnership matters.

- Each partner has different attributes which fit well together.

- The partners make a 'fair' investment proportional to their resources.

- There is a clear commitment to the partnership with respect to resources and the implementation of joint decisions.

- Individuals within the partnership have clearly stated responsibilities.

- The partners trust each other and are honest over partnership matters.

- The partners have open access to partnership information.

- The partners appreciate, respect and tolerate each others' differences.

- The partners offer each other mutual support.

- There is flexibility in accommodating partners' needs and views.

- The focus of the partnership working is a priority for both partners.

- The partners adapt their behaviour when undertaking joint working.

- There is a common understanding about language and communication.

- The risk/benefit balance is fair between the partners.

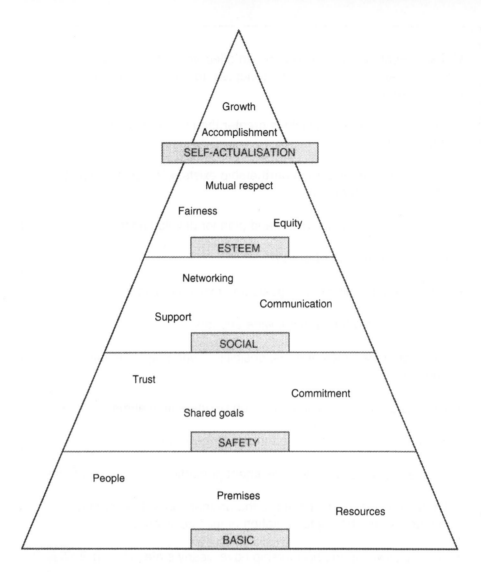

FIGURE Partnership hierarchy by Chambers (adapted from Maslow).[3]

EXERCISE 18   Review two of the three types of partnerships in which you are a participating partner against this checklist. Score a point for each feature that is present in your example of partnership and total them up.

1 You as a partner in the practice team, either with the other GPs or the practice staff.

2 Your practice and another organisation such as a local Trust or a voluntary organisation in the neighbourhood, or your primary care group.

3 You as a partner outside work with your spouse, a colleague, a sports partner or any other such partnership.

How many points did you score for the two examples? If very few, is there anything you can do to improve the partnership working? If you had high marks for both examples, are you in any other partnerships you might concentrate on?

- don't feel guilty about circumstances outside your control

EXERCISE 19   To what extent are you satisfied with your job overall?

- How satisfied are you overall with your job as a GP? *Usually very satisfied/Sometimes satisfied/Rarely or never satisfied.*

Review: If you are not generally satisfied with your current job in general practice or the mix of practice and other work, is there anything else you could do to enhance your job satisfaction? Could that include developing practice–patient relationships, developing another specialised professional interest, undertaking a new quality initiative or do other ideas appeal to you? Module 6 covers ideas for career development or even a career change. If you really are irreversibly dissatisfied with your current job, why not work through the next Module soon.

So what's your plan?

- smile and actively think positive thoughts

- look for the humour in a situation whenever appropriate

- seek out and encourage other positive people; avoid continual whingers

- value yourself for being assertive

- take pride in your achievements

- think future commitments through and visualise yourself positively in control

- make positive plans to learn from mistakes

- communicate confidently

- use positive body language.

Enhancing job satisfaction

MODULE 6
Promoting career development

AIMS

The aims of Module 6 are:

1 To improve awareness of general practice career options.

2 To increase GPs' understanding of the opportunities for career development.

3 To engage GPs in reflecting on their own career development to date.

4 To encourage GPs to actively plan the rest of their career.

CONTENTS

The total time to work through the module depends on the amount of time the reader spends reflecting on how the information in the module applies to him or her, before completing the exercises. The total time for which postgraduate education accreditation might be sought is four hours (including time for reading and reflecting and completing the exercises).*

---

* GP participants could apply to their region's Director of Postgraduate General Practice Education for permission to submit one or more completed modules for postgraduate education accreditation. Approval of such an application will be at the Director's discretion and may require the support of a local GP tutor in arranging assessment. No assessment will be undertaken by the author or Radcliffe Medical Press.

Here's what some GP participants at a career development course said about their experiences:

'The course had a great impact on me. A significant part of my life previously was my career ... the course has given me confidence in my personal abilities and my thinking and my decision making.'

'I am considering other career options in GP research and teaching.'

'The course ... broadened horizons within general practice, made me more keen ...'

'People set themselves up for failure and sabotage themselves in a million different ways.'

'Opened up my eyes to other opportunities I hadn't thought of before.'

'Gave me a jolt to realise in how limited a way I'd been thinking.'

STARTING TO THINK ABOUT CAREER DEVELOPMENT

You wouldn't be reading this workbook unless you were wondering if there is anything you can do to enhance or change your career. You may be just seeking reassurance that you are reasonably content in your current job, or alternatively wanting to review your whole career feeling that working in general practice is not for you. You may just want to check out what other opportunities there are. You may be finding that the other pressures in your life in combination with a busy life in general practice are just too much, whether that is through looking after young children or elderly dependents, or struggling to cope with physical or mental ill health, or other unsettling personal events.

This workbook should appeal to any GP wanting a career check-up. It should be useful for those established doctors who wonder if the grass is greener elsewhere or want to expand their horizons, those contemplating a career in general practice (students, young doctors), those in GP education who advise others about their career options, those with GP qualifications working as a GP non-principal or mainly outside general practice, and those who have personal reasons for wanting a mix of part-time work whilst looking after young children or coping with ill health.

Fulfilment and personal growth top Maslow's hierarchy of needs and are only likely to occur if the basics of an individual's life are in place – security, social networks, etc.[1] If you are contemplating a career change or expansion of your career that will require new skills, knowledge and experiences, you might be better waiting until your personal life is reasonably settled and you feel secure before making major alterations or moving on.

Medical students are often selected for their academic attainments rather than their personal qualities. The public seem to want the sort of doctors who take time and trouble to listen and empathise; but doctors who have the highest empathy levels with patients when tested as students and young junior housemen, are the ones who 10 years later have the least contact time with patients. Studies of doctors have found that an 'overly caring style' contributes to their heightened stress levels.[2,3] Some of these doctors, realising they cannot sustain the emotionally draining good doctor–patient relationships at which they excel full-time, reduce their general practice work and find alternative sessional work outside the practice to dilute the impact of their GP work.

GPs are often expected to conform to the traditional ways and styles of working of the practices they join. We should encourage doctors to dictate their own pace and styles at work and to encourage flexibility in their particular circumstances. Doctors who are forced to work faster than the pace they prefer not only become stressed but also underperform.[4]

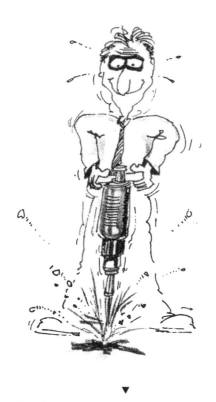

▼

Preparing the ground to make the most of your career.

The lack of a clear career structure is a well-recognised cause of stress in any workforce, not just medicine. To gauge the importance of this stress in medicine we have to remember the type of people who entered medical school. They were the 'achievers' at school, the ones who gained the top marks in the examinations and had that 'something extra' to persuade those interviewing for medical school that they would 'make the grade' as doctors. After a decade of striving and commitment they entered general practice to find high service demands and, all at once, a seeming dead end to their career, with no encouragement to continue studying and no recognition for improvements or further qualifications. Similarly, practice nurses can reach their top grade within several years of entering practice to find a flat career structure and no obvious route to promotion. NHS managers may think they have a career structure only to find that the NHS reorganisation changes are such that there is no obvious career progression and they need to transfer to a different pathway in another setting.

An additional stress for women doctors is that general practice may not have been their chosen career. Some women doctors leave the hospital specialty they would have preferred, such as paediatrics or obstetrics, because they see that few women make it to the top and that the general practice lifestyle is more likely to be compatible with bringing up a family. Even when they have become principals there is inequality between the sexes, with a tendency for male doctors to continue to manage the side of general practice looked upon as a traditionally masculine preserve, such as finance, computers and minor surgery, and female doctors concentrating on women's health in the practice. If you are not working in your chosen career specialty you are less likely to find your job satisfying and more likely to be stressed.

The BMA has followed up medical graduates from 1995 and found that the majority (71%) remained committed to the career they intended at graduation. Of the rest, 24% changed their career preference once within the three-year period following graduation and 4% changed more than once.[5]

Career planning

The key to career planning is information gathering from people, books and general observation. By conducting your career by chance rather than thoughtful planning you end up taking opportunities as they happen along, rather than taking control and finding the best match of career for your own needs and preferences.

It is difficult to plan your career and make informed choices about which specialty you will opt for with the sort of limited medical career counselling services that are available to medical students and qualified doctors, or if your experience of alternative medical specialties is limited.

Career planning is about career growth and the pathway along which you learn more about yourself, the facts about the options open to you, the implications of the alternative posts in terms of training, career progression, workload, etc., how to gain qualifications or fit yourself educationally for your preferred posts, how to manage the transition period whilst taking up new posts, and subsequently review and develop your career.

If you wish to switch careers or combine a substantial new post with your current GP job, you should plan ahead and go for a gradual transition rather than an impulsive change. Your previous experience should have paved the way for you to have a good understanding of the types of work and ways of working that suit you. The more the different components of your GP career overlap and you can carry your various skills and strengths over to the chosen post, the easier it is to break new ground from your relatively confident position.

All doctors need career planning at every stage of their careers. Many GPs still enjoy general practice, and there is the potential for retaining them in innovative ways with sabbaticals, new medical interests (e.g. inner-city developments), etc. Think positively well ahead of retirement age with financial planning, information about opportunities, enabling people to be creative in their career development. People are thinking of retiring earlier – the happiest people seem to be those who are enjoying the era of life in which they currently are. By the time they are 50 years old, people have more self-knowledge and are more aware of their boundaries, what makes them happy and satisfied, and how they like working, and can guard against what overloads or upsets them. So there's no need to be ageist; try and future-proof yourself against getting into a rut as you grow older. There are less changes in medicine than in many other organisations and professions, so you can keep up to date more easily than in professions such as computing. You may have less energy as you get older but your additional experience should make up for that, so there's no reason why someone in their fifties cannot perform as well if not better than a young doctor. You will have fewer financial and domestic pressures as the family grow up and leave home, and will be able to focus more on your work (if you want to!)

EXERCISE 1 Think back to reflect on how much of a role chance has played in your own career path.

How much is due to chance or an unexpected opportunity that you trained in medicine, or that you work in a primary care setting or your particular practice? Write your reflections down on how much was due to chance and whether there is any other job you might like to be doing now if you had planned your career differently:

On balance are you happy with your current career choice? *Yes/No*

If no, is it too late to change career track now, or could you combine your current job with another career activity related to the other choice of career? What do you think (be realistic!)?

Understanding your own career preferences and style

You cannot make a rational career choice without understanding the 'inner you' and what you have to offer. Your career and personality match are very important – and your personal preferences for the balance between work and leisure, work and income, degree of responsibility, type of work and extent of interaction with people.

There are many varieties of personality profile questionnaires. Two of the best known are the Myers Briggs type indicator,[6] which measures four bipolar dimensions of personality, and the 16PF questionnaire, which assesses 16 personality factors. In one *Return to General Practice* course for GP non-principals, most of the participants rated the workshop session where they received feedback on their Myers Briggs scores one of the best of the year's course. For many, becoming more aware of their personal preferences and styles meant that they gained confidence and pride in their own characteristics, rather than seeking to conform to a medical stereotype. Many thought that understanding themselves better would help them find practices where they were more likely to be compatible with the GP partners and practice character.

Although general practice offers a wide spectrum of opportunities which extend outside the traditional practice base, many doctors who wander too far away from their core specialty, general practice, eventually feel disconnected without their 'career anchor' of some direct contact with general practice.[7] They find they need to keep in touch and literally keep their hand in, and there are plenty of ex-GPs who have moved on to diverse jobs, such as medical advisers to health authorities, newspaper journalists or civil servants, who continue to do regular GP surgeries, not just for maintaining their credibility with their peers or keeping themselves up to date or their options for return open, but also to maintain their connection to their core career anchor in their lives.

Eight career anchor categories have been identified by Schein and used to increase people's insights about their strengths and motivation in career development: technical or functional competence; general managerial competence; autonomy or independence; security or stability; entrepreneurial creativity; service or dedication to a cause; pure challenge; lifestyle.[7] People define their self-image in terms of these traits and come to understand more about their talents, motives and values – and which of these is so important to them that they would not give up those facets of themselves if forced to make a choice.

EXERCISE 2   How well matched are you to your current job in primary care?

How well does your personality suit your current job? *Verywell/ Moderately/Not at all well*

What three key attributes about you personally match the requirements of your job (go on, sing your own praises, don't be humble):

-
-
-

What do you particularly like about the nature of your job, e.g. being with people, helping people, etc?

What is your 'career anchor', i.e. of the list described by Schein, above, what is the one feature about you and your job that you wouldn't give up, no matter what?

- technical or functional competence

- general managerial competence

- autonomy or independence

- security or stability

- entrepreneurial creativity

- service or dedication to a cause

- pure challenge

- lifestyle.

Gaining medical careers information, advice, guidance or counselling

Careers guidance, advice and help resources in England and Wales are patchy, and few junior doctors, general practitioner registrars, principals and non-principals have access to well-informed, impartial general practice careers advisers.[8] In hospital practice, careers advice and guidance is usually provided by clinical tutors of particular specialties, but comprehensive careers counselling that gives an overview of all specialties and in-depth help to doctors with particular problems is lacking.

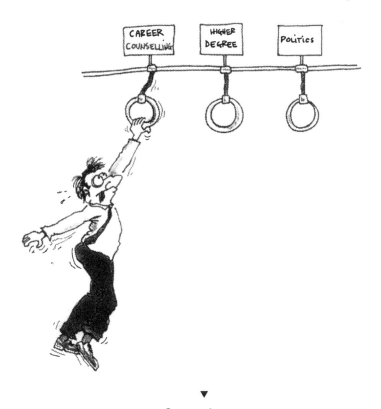

▼

Career change.

To make a rational career choice you need *careers information,* giving you the facts. That is, the provision of written and/or verbal information about career opportunities, including the number and type of posts available at a particular level and in a particular specialty, and details of the qualifications and training necessary. *Careers guidance* is more personal and directive, and provides advice within the context of the opportunities that are available. It is useful for those who have not made a career decision or who have decided on their career goal but are unaware of the best way of achieving it. *Careers counselling* is a more intensive process, requiring specialist skills. Ideally, careers counselling builds on careers advice or guidance, appraisal and assessment, and pastoral support. It includes the recognition and analysis of a person's strengths and weaknesses with respect to available career options. Careers counselling involves a facilitatory approach for students or doctors uncertain of their career direction or who have particular career problems, such as those who have a health disability or whose career is constrained by personal circumstances or who seem unsuited to their current post.[9]

Established doctors wanting to change their career direction may require careers information, careers guidance, careers counselling or personal counselling depending on their individual circumstances and how far along they are with career planning.

Effective medical careers services should be 'available, accessible, appropriate, accurate, impartial, confidential, performed by people who have been trained to do it, and responsive to culture and gender', according to the BMA.[10] For most doctors the sort of careers advice they have received, if any, has been the 'Be like me' kind, with senior doctors describing their own careers as role models to be followed.

Doctors who are born with or develop a disability experience discrimination at work, where colleagues are reluctant to accommodate their special needs, and problems with medical education held in venues with poor access for the disabled. The NHS cannot afford to continue to maintain such negative attitudes to disabled doctors, not only because the NHS should be acting as a good role model to other organisations in optimising the working potential of those with disabilities, but also because of the current threat to GP workforce numbers in many areas of the UK. Targeted help and support might increase the numbers who stay in active medical practice for longer, whether it be doctors who have become disabled by stress and other mental ill-health problems or who are physically disabled or suffering from chronic ill health.

EXERCISE 3   Do you know where you could obtain careers information, advice, guidance or counselling?

Think back – have you ever received such help? *Yes/No*

If so was it from someone who was experienced, who was well informed and gave impartial advice, and who had dedicated time to spend with you?

Do you know where to get such information, advice or counselling from? Does your local higher education college have generic careers advisers who you might see, or might they advise you where other professional career advice is available?

FLEXIBLE WORKING

Could you take a more flexible approach to general practice working?

Flexible working may be a good way of counteracting burnout by enabling the doctor to pursue other interests and keep their creativity and enjoyment of general practice alive if working day after day in the surgery is debilitating or a problem. Some doctors just want to earn extra money by taking on additional work outside their core job, whilst others are keeping their options open with a variety of jobs until they focus down sometime in the future.

Flexible working is being seen as one way of solving the looming crisis in GP numbers, by increasing the attractiveness of general practice and retaining doctors who might otherwise be put off entering general practice or looking for a full partnership and risking investing in expensive surgery premises. Similarly, flexible working in nursing and other primary care professions retains staff who might otherwise not be able to work due to family commitments.

Flexibility is essential if doctors are to adapt to change. Much stress arises in general practice when people resist change and blindly persist with the same traditional systems and ways of working in a time warp. Society is constantly changing, demands and possibilities are very different, and new ways of working are necessary if those working in general practice are to flourish and survive. The UK workforce as a whole is more mobile, and more married women have paid jobs than used to. Working wives still do much more housework than husbands.[11]

One of the main stimuli to increasing the flexibility of working arrangements has been the increased proportion of women coming into general practice, as GP partners, assistants or retainees, or as practice nurses. Women GP registrars outnumber men, and women make up 27% of the whole time equivalent workforce, a rise of 4% since 1991.[12] There has been a trend to part-time working by male GPs as well as women doctors, as the box shows.

BOX

- Trend to part-time GP working (95% full-time in 1990, 85% full-time in 1997)

- Falling full-time female GP trend (84% full-time 1990, 63% full-time 1997)

- Rising number female GP job sharers (3% in 1990, 5% in 1997)

- Rising number half-time female GPs (2% in 1990, 14% in 1997)

- Rising number three-quarters time female GPs (11% in 1990, 18% in 1997)

- Rising number part-time [half or three-quarters time] male GPs (2% in 1990, 5% in 1997)

Types of flexible working

The strengths of a portfolio career are the flexibility, variety, personal development and ability to react to new opportunities or changing circumstances – either your personal ones or in relation to the NHS organisation. It is much better to seize the opportunities whilst you are on top of your job and starting to need variety and new challenges, rather than waiting until you are starting to burn out from the constant workload of being a long-term GP. It's all about choice – working additional overnight shifts for a GP co-operative with a subsequent day off funded by employing a regular GP assistant involves calculating the balance between benefits and disadvantages for you as an individual and you as a practice.

Flexible working patterns require flexibility from GP partners or employers as much as the doctor concerned. The success of any innovative working arrangement depends as much on the willingness and attitudes of everyone involved as on the structure put in place as a framework to accommodate that work.

Job sharing

The popularity of job sharing is slowly increasing such that 5% of male and female GPs have made this type of arrangement. This normally involves two people sharing one full-time post, usually but not necessarily with a 50:50 split of hours, tasks and pay. Two job sharer GPs must receive at least one third of the income of the highest earning partner between them, although this may be divided unequally between the two sharers. Such job-sharing posts often come as a way of a full-time postholder reducing his or her hours for personal or professional reasons, but sometimes a pair of doctors or other health professionals submit a joint application for an advertised vacancy and convince the interview panel that 'two heads are better than one'. Many regional offices of the BMA or health authorities will help doctors seeking potential job-share partners and hold personal details on a database. Some job-share partners divide the week in half, others do half of each day. Sometimes job sharers deputise for each other over holiday or sickness absence periods. Many have a period of overlap at least once a week to allow them to pass messages and communicate, some working closely as a pair sharing the management of individual patients and others acting as any other partner would. There is resistance to job sharing in some partnerships by those who think that job sharing means a lack of continuity of care, that extra doctors confuse the patients, who worry about filling half a shared post if one partner leaves and the additional costs of practice infrastructure, and any financial penalties from receiving one set of allowances from one shared post as opposed to two separate part-time posts. If one job-share partner leaves, a practice has six months to replace them before the job-share approval lapses when the remaining share partner will have to become a part-time or full-time partner. But the benefits seem to exceed the drawbacks in the majority of job-sharing arrangements which enable doctors working part-time to be principals rather than assistants, to combine the full responsibilities of a being a partner with others outside work.

Retainer scheme

There are around 600 to 700 doctors on the retainer scheme in the UK, about 90% of whom are in general practice. Most are women doctors. Since June 1998, GP practices employing assistants for up to four sessions per week are entitled to an allowance of £45.75 for every 3.5 hour half-day session. A doctor can remain as a retainer for a maximum of five years. The retainer fee is currently £300 pa (to cover some of the costs of membership of a Defence Union and subscribing to a professional journal). Practices employing retainees need not be training practices, but must be capable of providing adequate education, supervision and support.

Salaried doctors

Salaried GP options can co-exist with a self-employed GP service. But there is a risk of the salaried doctor being exploited – and many have left or avoided salaried positions in the past because of being asked to do maximal work for minimal pay. There is a whole variety of salaried positions, although they are still few and far between. More are springing up tailored to local needs, such as through Primary Care Act Pilots or Personal Medical Services Pilots where salaried doctors are employed with a specific remit, such as providing extra care for the homeless, or relieving inner-city GPs practising in areas where it is more difficult to recruit GP principals. Primary care groups may consider sharing salaried GPs between practices to help with sickness or holiday cover. Associate schemes exist to provide relief for single-handed GPs in remote areas.

Flexible training

The UK does offer a limited number of flexible training placements for a variety of specialties. Part-time training is at least a half-time commitment under European Law. The UK is one of only two European countries with an undersupply of doctors (–0.9% medical unemployment) and this, the long training periods in the UK and the relatively high population to doctor ratios in the UK have fuelled the need to establish flexible training schemes

---

to retain as many doctors as possible. General practice offers great opportunities for creative ways to accommodate doctors with special needs regarding part-time training, for example those with pressing domestic responsibilities or disabilities. As GP registrars are supernumerary their training can focus on more study periods, their hours can be organised to ease child care with a concentration during school hours or during the 5 to 8pm 'twilight' shift when there may be someone else available to care for the children or other dependents.

There are many postgraduate educational qualifications for which the training is part-time and can be theoretically fitted in around work, although in reality this usually swallows up a lot of family time and annual leave and requires considerable drive and commitment to succeed. Examples of the types of qualifications that can lead on to other job opportunities are given below:

- Diploma in Occupational Health either by distance learning or in residential blocks

- Masters or Diploma in Sports Medicine

- Masters of Business Affairs (MBA) or a Diploma

- Masters in Education

- Diploma in Prison Medicine

- Complementary medicine qualification such as in acupuncture or homeopathy

- Non-medical qualification

- Doctorate (MD or DM) or other research degree.

Portfolio medical careers

This is just the fashionable term ascribed to mixing and matching different posts, usually centring on healthcare in some way; some people successfully run medical and non-medical jobs together, but usually one complements or feeds off the others. The *portfolio* description implies that the skills involved in the mix of jobs are transferable and can be carried on afterwards to the next sequence of jobs the individual health professional takes on.

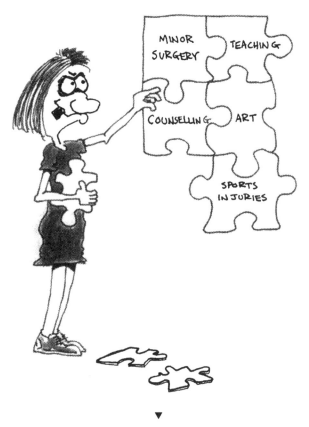

▼

Portfolio careers.

Disadvantages of flexible working

A major barrier to flexible working is the attitude of other GPs who scorn the part-timer or assistant for not being a 'proper' GP and shirking full responsibility. There is a lack of understanding from peers as well as the public/patients about doctors and other health professionals working less than full time. Work colleagues may be suspicious of you because you are different and challenge their choice of long-stay posts. Some voice concerns that if too many GPs change to flexible working, mixing and matching various posts or specifying that they will only work between 9am and 5pm, there may be too few full-time doctors left as the mainstay GPs of a practice to cover the antisocial hours and routine or behind the scenes work.

Many of those working in minimally part-time posts feel isolated within their practices, especially if their working hours mean that coffee breaks and practice meetings do not coincide with when the others are free. Isolation is an issue for someone who is only one of a kind in a practice or other workplace setting, and some protected release to group education with peers can guard against isolation.

Financial penalties are often what drive freelance doctors to find a secure source of income through partnerships or long-term assistantships or employed posts. The financial insecurity from the lack of an NHS pension or sickness cover and the drain of constantly looking for work and keeping financial records take their toll and sap energy. Pay is usually relatively lower as a locum or casual worker compared with being in a permanent position or being a principal when the locum's lack of income whilst on holiday, sick or training is taken into account.

Limited IT skills can be a factor in making life difficult for doctors or nurses moving between paperless practices with varied computer systems and no instructions. This also restricts access to electronic databases of best practice or even locum and partnership vacancies.

In some practices all income earned outside the practice is pooled by the GP partners. It is usual that external work done during normal working hours is paid into the practice account as shared income, as the other partners will be covering for the absent GP by seeing extra patients in surgery, taking additional home visits and dealing with the general practice workload. Many practices have different financial arrangements such that individual GPs keep externally earned pay for work done completely outside normal working hours in their own time, so long as the additional work does not impinge on the practice such as it would if one of the GPs worked as a casualty officer through the night and fell asleep at their desk the next morning.

Another drawback that is rarely realised until after the change to a flexible working arrangement has been made and the doctor is spending more time outside the practice, is the effect that his or her lesser availability has on patients who are used to being able to consult them in person or on the phone relatively easily. Patients who regard doctor X as being *their* doctor get fed up if he or she is often away and they are faced with a constantly changing sea of doctors standing in for doctor X. Their disaffection creates guilt and regret in doctors who had previously taken the 'continuity of care' they provided for granted.

One other aspect you should consider is what effects a new working environment may have on you and if they are acceptable. Doctors who branch out from general practice to take on a part-time educational post seem to remain rooted in general practice, but those who take up management positions, especially full-time positions, are often influenced by management thinking and behaviour to the extent that their GP colleagues may feel estranged and accuse them of having lost their GP persona. Sometimes clinicians turned managers embrace their new found management philosophy with such zeal that they outdo any died in the wool manager for getting GPs' prescribing costs down or other performance measure achieved.

CAREER OPTIONS

The spectrum of GP-related posts is vast and covers the following categories:

Education

Posts include the pyramid structure from being a GP trainer in a training practice, a course organiser for GP registrars on a vocational training scheme, an educational facilitator for GP non-principals, a GP lecturer in a university department of general practice for undergraduate medical students or postgraduate doctors and other health professionals, a GP tutor to medical students in your practice, or perhaps a GP mentor on a postgraduate educational project.

If you want more information about these posts contact the Director of General Practice Postgraduate Education in your region, the Dean or Professor of your local university Department of General Practice or Primary Care, or contact anyone in these posts to find out more.

Service posts

These type of posts include clinical assistant posts, assistants at specialised clinics such as for the homeless, visiting GPs to prisons, family planning doctors, school medical officers (each school has different requirements involving mix of sessional work, surgeries, on call and varying responsibilities from usual GMS, health promotion, medical assessments of new pupils, etc.), a military cadetship (available to medical students during their last three years of training in the army, navy and airforce who go on to take up a six year commission) or territorial army place, GP co-operatives or deputising agencies and medical locums (not necessarily GP ones), Benefits Agency sessions, occupational health sessions for the NHS or a private company.

Information is available from whoever is responsible for the service, through adverts in professional journals or the 'grapevine'.

Advisory

Posts include giving expert or specialised medical advice to health authorities, patients' organisations, the Department of Health, assisting medical defence organisations, pharmaceutical companies, computing or other commercial companies who want a healthcare or GP opinion and input, such as in making video films destined to be viewed by other GPs.

Information about opportunities is available from those who want the advice or via the grapevine. Some posts are widely advertised in local and national newspapers, particularly those on public bodies that operate under the 'Nolan' rules of fair behaviour, such as non-executive directors of NHS Trust Boards or NHS advisory committees.

Research

Alternative ways to develop an academic career might be:

- Being a research fellow, research assistant, lecturer at undergraduate medical school or postgraduate medical school or School of Health. You may be able to combine doing a job in a specific post and working for a higher degree in parallel.

- Gaining a training fellowship, for example an RCGP research fellowship or NHS regional training fellowship supervised by an academic unit. You would combine your GP job with protected time for research and undertake a higher degree attached to a supervisory academic unit.

- Registering for a higher degree (MPhil, PhD, MD) with a view to gaining an academic appointment when you have obtained the research qualification.

- Joining a GP research network run by an academic unit and participating in the data collection or analysis/interpretative stage of a project, for which you may or may not be paid.
- Joining a research general practice which receives some regional funding for protected time and infrastructure; but these are few and far between.

Academic success is judged on the numbers and quality (journal of publication) of peer-reviewed publications, numbers, sources, magnitude of research grants gained, national recognition, such as presentations at conferences, peer reviewers, expert committees.

There are considerable difficulties in pursuing an academic career. These include less pay than in a service post, opportunities are not always advertised, levels of departmental support are variable, the relatively low status of academic GPs, the limited time for academic research and education work in service general practice, the exorbitant costs of registration for a higher postgraduate degree and scarcity of funds for small research projects.

Communications

These posts include writing for professional medical journals, for the lay press or books. GPs might join the GP Writers Association or Media Medics if they want to join a network of other writers. The annual *Writers Handbook* gives contact details for a variety of publications, describing which accept unsolicited material and their pay scales. Contacting the editor is usually the first step and tempting them to look at your exciting outline or ideas for article(s).

Speaking on the radio and TV can be time-consuming and may attract little or no pay, but can increase your profile and open the way to other work or career opportunities.

Medico-political

These include posts on the Local Medical Committee and as their representative at regional level or the national General Practice Committee, or as an officer on the national primary care management organisations. Most positions do not attract direct pay but do reimburse some expenses, including locum fees.

Elections are held periodically. You are more likely to succeed if you hold other relevant appointments.

Medico-legal

Insurance companies are often on the lookout for dependable GPs who will see clients and write reports promptly and provide an expert opinion on an ongoing claim. Other posts include working for the police as a police surgeon or expert, such as in sexual assault cases. A disadvantage can be the time spent in court if claims are contested.

Commercial or business

Besides those mentioned under the advisory posts section, you might start your own company by extending a hobby or skill such as computing or a non-medical interest such as travel. Sports medicine, information technology and complementary medicine are all potentially good fields for starting new businesses.

Management

A common option is to combine general practice with management in PCGs, with trusts, health authorities, Medical Audit Advisory Groups, etc. There seems to be a blurred boundary between chairing and managing a body which is often dependent on the extent of the infrastructure of that body and how much work can be delegated.

EXERCISE 5   Which of the alternative medical career areas described above appeal to you?

Does any job described in this section appeal to you? *Yes/No*

If so, how long have you been thinking of getting involved in that area?

What is stopping you finding out about opportunities or taking up such a post?

Pros and cons of taking on a job outside the practice

Besides the financial incentive, you will learn a lot about a different branch of medicine or from the new people you meet in the course of the additional post. It is easy to get bogged down in the day-to-day stresses and demands of general practice or oppressed by the more mundane parts, and breaking out into new territory helps to keep the practice in perspective and yourself fresh. Getting outside the practice and working with other professionals you wouldn't normally meet gives you a broader perspective of medicine and life in general.

You will need to make an honest assessment of why you should opt for a particular post. The effort involved in meeting the skills and responsibilities of the new post will probably be considerable and should not just be undertaken because it happens to be available and you are flattered that someone has asked you to apply. If you foresee a good opportunity for personal development and the potential job interests you, you might decide that the pay is of secondary importance.

The more skills you have the more marketable you are and the more you can dictate your pay and conditions. But you may need assertiveness skills to make sure that others offering the post understand the skills, knowledge and experience you will be bringing and to negotiate a good rate of pay. If you think that by undertaking a job you will become better known in the area or that it will subsequently attract extra work or custom, you may choose to do the initial job for little or no pay. But don't let people assume you'll do a job free, only do so by your choice.

Find a buddy, mentor, co-tutor or coach

You have made a good start by working through this workbook and reassessing your career and how satisfied you are with different aspects of it. You will be more likely to follow your action plans and overcome hiccups in your progress if you have a trusted friend or adviser with whom to discuss your career path.

You might ask a friend who is a GP in another practice whom you meet regularly if you can listen to each other, give practical or emotional support, swop information and identify possible solutions. An equal relationship between you might be described as a buddy, a co-tutor or peer supporter.

A mentor relationship would be a more one-way relationship where the mentor had the time and capacity to listen to you and help facilitate you making decisions about your career. Some educational mentors are only concerned with helping the doctor being mentored identify and meet their educational or training needs through a development plan, whereas others might give practical or emotional support too. A regular appraisal of your career once a year by someone who is interested and whose opinion you respect is a great way to boost your morale and motivation.

A coach could offer more directive help about your career in the same way that a sports coach urges an athlete on. Coaching involves training, supporting, instructing and motivating others to improve their performance by a working partnership between client and coach to achieve agreed goals. A good coach is said to have psychology, business and communication skills. Coaches work through one-to-one conversations in person or by email.

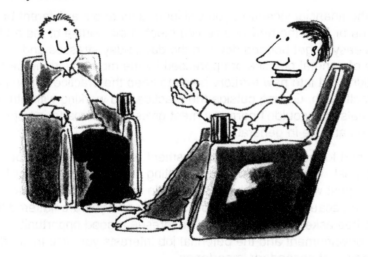

▼

'Buddies'.

EXERCISE 6   Who could you discuss your career development with?

Now that you've read some suggestions about finding someone with whom to discuss your career progress or aspirations, you should think out how that applies to you. What kind of confidant might suit you, e.g. GP tutor, non-medical careers adviser, a buddy?

Have you any particular person in mind whom you might engage in such a relationship?

Write down at least three topics that you would like to discuss in this way, e.g. possibilities for career development.

And finally

EXERCISE 7   Reassess your current job by summarising the positive and negative factors relating to your current job and making a timetabled action plan for taking your career forward.

The positive factors will include the good bits of your job, what makes it worthwhile and why you do it; the negative factors will include the down side of your job and what you would change if you could.

Positives:

Negatives:

How does the positive side compare with the negative side? *Positive side outweighs the negative side/About equal/Negative side outweighs the positive side.*

Continued

Do you want to make changes, e.g. change your current job, change to a different way of working?

What are your new goals?

What actions will you take to achieve your goals, e.g. gain new skills, look at advertisements, undertake personality assessment, etc? Who can help? When?

•

•

•

•

•

When will you review your progress with your career development?

References

1 Maslow AH (1970) *Motivation and personality.* Harper and Row, New York.

2 Firth-Cozens J (1997) Predicting stress in general practitioners: 10 year follow up postal survey. *BMJ.* **315**: 34–5.

3 Firth-Cozens J (1998) Individual and organisational predictors of depression in general practitioners. *Br J Gen Pract.* **48**: 1647–51.

4 Howie J, Porter A, Heaney D, Hopton J (1991) Long to short consultation ratio: a proxy measure of quality of care for general practice. *Br J Gen Pract.* **41**: 48–54.

5 British Medical Association (1998) *Cohort study. Third report, June 1998. Career intentions of first year senior house officers.* Health policy and Economic Research Unit, BMA.

6 Myers Briggs I, Myers P (1996) *Gifts differing: understanding personality type.* Davies-Black Publishing, California.

7 Schein E (1990) *Career anchors: discovering your real needs.* Pfeiffer and Co, Oxford.

8 Chambers R (1995) *Careers in general practice: towards a more informed choice. Availability of career guidance for general practice in England and Wales in 1995.* An RCGP Revaluing General Practice Initiative, Keele University.

9 Percy D, Temple J (1998) *Department of Health SHO implementation Working Group. Provision of careers counselling.* Letter to Royal Colleges, 31 July 1998 (adapted).

10 British Medical Association (1996) *Guidelines for the provision of careers services for doctors.* British Medical Association, London.

11 Gershuny J, Berthoud R (1997) *New partnerships? Men and women in the 1990s.* ESRC Research Centre on Micro-social Change. University of Essex.

12 Department of Health (1998) *Statistics for general medical practitioners 1987–1997.* Bulletin 1998/16. DoH, London.

RESOURCES

Books and information leaflets

Allen I (1988) *Any room at the top? A study of doctors and their careers.* Policy Studies Institute, London.

Allen I (1994) *Doctors and their careers.* Policy Studies Institute, London.

Anderson C (1996) *How to organise a careers forum for general practice.* University of Nottingham, Nottingham.

Anderson C, Turner R (1998) *Career handbook for medical students.* University of Nottingham, Nottingham.

Army Medical Services (1998) *Career opportunities for soldiers and officers: challenging careers in the medical, dental, veterinary and nursing professions.* Army Recruiting Group, London.

Booher D (1997) *Get ahead, stay ahead! Learn the 70 most important career skills, traits and attitudes to: stay employed, get promoted, get a better job.* McGraw-Hill, London.

Briggs Myers I, Myers P (1980) *Gifts differing: understanding personality types.* Davies-Black publishing, California.

British Medical Association (1994) *Guidelines for good practice in the recruitment and selection of doctors.* Career Progress of Doctors Committee, BMA, London.

British Medical Association (1997) *Medical careers: a general guide.* BMA, London. Also *Guidance note supplement: useful addresses.* BMA (1997).

British Medical Association (1996) *Guidelines for the provision of careers services for doctors.* BMA, London.

British Medical Association (1998) *Doctors' pay*. BMA, London. (Describes pay structures and pay levels for various branches of the profession and other employed posts, such as police surgeon, armed forces doctors, deputising doctors.)

Eggert M (1992) *The perfect cv: all you need to get it right first time*. Arrow Business books, London.

Francis D (1994) *Managing your own career*. Harper Collins, London.

Handy C (1995) *The age of unreason*. Arrow Business books, London.

Johnson C, Forrest F, Hall C (1998) *Getting ahead in medicine*. BIOS Scientific Publishers, Oxford.

Kent S (1997) *Creating your own career: practical advice for graduates in a changing world*. Kogan Page, London.

Leider R (1994) *Life skills: taking charge of your personal and professional growth*. Pfeiffer and Co, London.

McKenna F, Pickersgill D (eds) (1995) *The GP's guide to professional and private work outside the NHS*. Radcliffe Medical Press, Oxford.

Morrell J, Roberts A (1995) Make an application for flexible (part time) training. *BMJ.* **311**: 242–4.

Nelson Bolles R (1996) *What colour is your parachute? A practical manual for job hunters and career changers*. Ten Speed Press, California.

NHS Executive (1996) *Making your choice in medicine*. NHSE, Leeds.

Norfolk Health Authority (1993) *Job sharing in general practice*. Human Resources Department, Norfolk Health Authority.

Pemberton C, Refause J, Evans C (1998) *Managing career dilemmas*. Financial Times Management, London.

Petchey R, Williams J, Baker M (1996) *Junior doctors, medical careers and general practice*. University of Nottingham, Nottingham.

Royal College of General Practitioners (1997) *Information Sheet Number 18. Additional career options in general practice*. RCGP, London.

Royal College of General Practitioners (1996) *Information Sheet Number 14. Women general practitioners*. RCGP, London.

Schein E (1990) *Career anchors: discovering your real needs*. Pfeiffer and Co, Oxford.

Schein E (1990) *Career anchors: trainer's manual*. Pfeiffer and Co, Oxford.

Turner B (ed) (1998) *The writer's handbook 1998*. Macmillan, Basingstoke.

Ward C, Eccles S (1997) *So you want to be a brain surgeon? A medical careers guide*. Oxford Medical Publications, Oxford.

Women in Medicine (1998) *Careers for women in medicine: planning and pitfalls*. Women in Medicine Collective.

Women in Medicine (1998) *Job-sharing and part-time work in general practice (booklet)*. Women in Medicine.

Courses: examples

GP tutor Dr Ian Sidford in Redditch brings out an annual booklet describing part-time and distance learning degree, diploma, certificate, PGEA and other courses for medical practitioners in the UK. Contact: Mrs Lee Sidford, 44 Salop Road, Redditch, Worcs B97 4PS.

Ashridge Development Programmes for Executives. Ashridge is an international centre for management and organisation development. Courses range from short day programmes in strategic management, leadership, performance and personal skills to one-year full-time or several years part-time MBA or general manager programmes. Contact: Ashridge Management College, Berkhamsted, Hertfordshire HP4 1NS. Email:*info@ashridge.org.uk*

Centre for Health Planning and Management, University of Keele runs senior management programmes, the diploma in management for doctors, full- and part-time MBA (Health Executive) programme. Contact: Darwin Building, University of Keele, Keele, Staffs ST5 5BG. Fax: 01782 711737

Diploma in Occupational Medicine. The Institute of Occupational Health at the University of Birmingham offers a three-part course covering the syllabus for the Diploma examination of the Faculty of Occupational Medicine, Royal College of Physicians. The Distance Learning Unit of the Centre for Occupational Health at the University of Manchester also runs a Diploma course, as do several other universities.

Health Services Management Centre, University of Birmingham runs leadership and management development programmes for senior managers and clinicians in the NHS as well as a range of targeted short courses. Internet: *http://www.bham.ac.uk/hsmc/* Contact: Park House, 40 Edgbaston Park Road, Birmingham B15 2RT.

Health Services Management Unit, University of Manchester. NHS management development programmes. Contact: Devonshire House, University Precinct Centre, Oxford Road, Manchester M13 9PL. Fax: 0161 273 5245.

Institute of Health and Care Development. IHCD runs career development programmes and undertakes consultancy on organisational development issues. It is supported by the NHS Executive and provides the officially endorsed Career Management Programmes for mid-career NHS staff in England. Contact: IHCD, St Bartholomews Court, 18 Christmas Street, Bristol BS1 5BT. Internet: *http://www.ihcd.org.uk* Tel: 0117 929 1029.

King's Fund Management College. Programmes for general management, personal and professional development, and leadership aimed at improving the clinical, professional and managerial ledership of the NHS. Internet: *http://www.kingsfund.org,uk*. Contact: 11–13 Cavendish Square, London W1M 0AN. Tel: 0171 307 2400.

Open University Business School runs management development programmes including MBA. Centre for Higher Education Practice in the Open University runs the postgraduate certificate in teaching and learning in higher education and other higher education courses. Contact: The Open University, Milton Keynes MK7 6AA Internet: *http://cehep.open.ac.uk* Fax: 01908 858438.

Organisations

British Association of Medical Managers (BAMM). Barnes Hospital, Kingsway, Cheadle, Cheshire SK8 2NY. Fax: 0161 491 4254. BAMM organises management and leadership development programmes, and conferences, and supports members.

Career Dilemmas Forum has set up a network to support organisations and individuals overcome specific career dilemmas by giving practical help. It offers coaching and mentoring support, careers counselling skills training, careers workshops and self-development support programmes. The Corm House, Tathall End, Hanslope, Bucks MK19 7NF.

Career Management Service. A programme for NHS professionals. It offers a service for individuals who aspire to senior posts in the NHS who want to maximise their performance and job satisfaction in their present posts via personal development plans. Career Management, St Bartholomews Court, 18 Christmas Street, Bristol BS1 5BT. Fax: 0117 925 0574.

Career Track International supplies seminars and audio and videotapes on management and leadership skills, appraisal, team building, stress management, delegation, mastering change, motivation, computing and personal skills such as building self-esteem. Career Track International, Sunrise House, Sunrise Parkway, Linford Wood, Milton Keynes MK14 6YA. Internet: *http://www.careertrack.com* Tel: 01908 354101 (tapes); 01908 354000 (seminars).

General Practice Writers Association. Membership details from The General Secretary, GPWA, 633 Liverpool Road, Southport, Merseyside PR8 3NG. Tel: 01704 577839.

Institute of Personnel and Development (IPD). A European organisation that deals with the management and development of people. The publications and training packs offer educational resources in these fields. Distributors: Plymbridge Distributors Ltd, Estover, Plymouth PL6 7PZ. Internet: *http://www.ipd.co.uk*

Media Medics. Dr Paul Stillman, Claybrooke, Haywards, Pound Hill, Crawley, Sussex RH10 3TR. Tel: 01293 889100; Fax: 01293 882100.

Medical Forum offers independent career guidance and personal development for health career professionals, in person, as small group workshops and by email career coaching. Director: Dr Sonia Hutton-Taylor, Greyhound House, Richmond TW9 1HY. Fax: 01256 773226/07020 933964. Internet: *http://fast.to/medicalforum*

Medical Officers of Schools Association (MOSA) issues guideline fee scales. C/o Amherst Medical Practice, 21 St Botolph's Road, Sevenoaks, Kent TN13 3AQ.

Medical Women's Federation has careers advisers in each NHS region in England, Wales and Scotland. MWF, BMA House, Tavistock Square, London WC1H 9JP.

NHS Senior Career Development Service/Executive Choice. This is run by Dearden Management in association with the Health Services Management Unit at the University of Manchester. The service is aimed at managers and clinicians working just below Board level. It offers careers counselling and coaching, training, briefing and networking. Membership includes a regular newsletter, access to masterclasses on personal and professional development skills and coaching. Executive Choice, Dearden Management, Church Road, Redhill, Bristol BS18 7SG. Fax: 01934 863390. Internet: *http://www.nhs-ExecChoice.co.uk*

UK Register of Expert Witnesses. C/o Debby Dyson, at JS Publications, PO Box 505, Newmarket, Suffolk CB8 7TF.

Women in Medicine. An organisation of women doctors and medical students founded in 1981. Provides a forum for discussion and a campaigning voice as well as acting as a support network. Runs local support groups, an annual conference and a bi-monthly newsletter. 21 Wallingford Avenue, London W10 6QA.